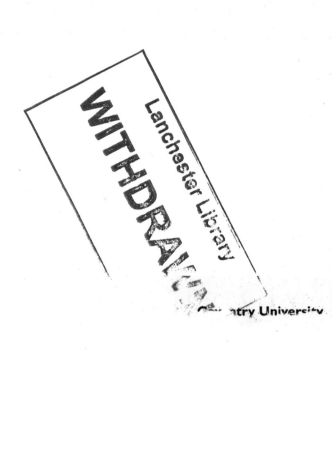

Neuroanatomy

AN ILLUSTRATED COLOUR TEXT

For Elsevier Churchill Livingstone

Commissioning Editor: Timothy Horne
Project Development Manager: Helen Leng
Project Manager: Nancy Arnott
Designer: Erik Bigland
Illustration Manager: Bruce Hogarth
First and second editions illustrated by Raymond
Evans, Denise Smith and Caroline Wilkinson,
Unit of Art in Medicine, School of Biological
Sciences, The University of Manchester
Third edition illustrated by PCA Creative, Ethan
Danielson and Bruce Hogarth

Neuroanatomy

AN ILLUSTRATED COLOUR TEXT | THIRD EDITION

A R Crossman PhD DSc
Professor of Anatomy
Faculty of Life Sciences
The University of Manchester
Manchester, UK

D Neary MD FRCP
Professor of Neurology
The University of Manchester
Manchester, UK

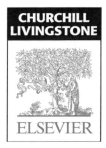

CHURCHILL LIVINGSTONE

ELSEVIER

EDINBURGH   LONDON   NEW YORK   OXFORD   PHILADELPHIA   ST LOUIS   SYDNEY   TORONTO   2005

ELSEVIER CHURCHILL LIVINGSTONE
An imprint of Elsevier Limited

First edition 1995
Second edition 2000
Third edition 2005

ISBN 0-443-10036-5

British Library Cataloguing in Publication Data
A catalogue record for this book is available from the British Library

Library of Congress Cataloging in Publication Data
A catalog record for this book is available from the Library of Congress

Note
Medical knowledge is constantly changing. Standard safety
precautions must be followed, but as new research and clinical
experience broaden our knowledge, changes in treatment and drug
therapy may become necessary or appropriate. Readers are advised to
check the most current product information provided by the
manufacturer of each drug to be administered to verify the
recommended dose, the method and duration of administration, and
contraindications. It is the responsibility of the practitioner, relying on
experience and knowledge of the patient, to determine dosages and
the best treatment for each individual patient. Neither the publisher
nor the authors assumes any liability for any injury and/or damage to
persons or property arising from this publication.

The Publisher

ELSEVIER SCIENCE your source for books,
journals and multimedia
in the health sciences
www.elsevierhealth.com

Working together to grow
libraries in developing countries

www.elsevier.com | www.bookaid.org | www.sabre.org

ELSEVIER   BOOK AID International   Sabre Foundation

The
publisher's
policy is to use
**paper manufactured
from sustainable forests**

Printed in Spain

Preface to the Third Edition

The principal aim of this, like each previous, edition of *Neuroanatomy* is to provide students of medicine and science with a clear, concise, well-organised and visually attractive account of the anatomy of the human nervous system. Neuroanatomy remains a fundamental cornerstone for the understanding of nervous system function and dysfunction. Over recent years, however, in many medical schools, the time in the undergraduate medical curriculum devoted to instruction in anatomy has been progressively eroded. Since neuroanatomy is often regarded by students as the most difficult area of anatomy to grasp, we believe that now more than ever there is a need for a focused and succinct undergraduate text which presents the relevant material in sufficient detail to enable understanding of how the nervous system works and to provide the basis for the diagnosis and treatment of neurological conditions.

A number of improvements and revisions have been included in the new edition whilst at the same time every effort has been made not to increase the length of the book significantly. The first chapter has been further developed to provide an expanded overview of the entire topic including the basic neuroanatomical principles, the main sensory, motor and cognitive systems, and the fundamentals of clinical diagnosis of neurological disease. A new chapter has been included (Chapter 17) in which a number of common neurological clinical scenarios are presented; in each case the syndrome described, the anatomical site of the lesion and the diagnosis can be found within the pages of the book (the answers also being provided). It is intended that students following the currently popular 'problem-based' curricula will find these cases helpful and that all enquiring students will find the solving of these clinical puzzles a satisfying experience.

Manchester   A R Crossman
2004   D Neary

Preface to the First Edition

This book has been written primarily for undergraduate medical students. At the same time, we have borne in mind students following other health science courses where a basic understanding of the nervous system and its major disorders is required, and also students of basic neuroscience, who are invariably intrigued and edified by discussion of the disorders which afflict the human nervous system.

The book has been prepared during a period of widespread debate on, and evolution in, the substance and style of medical education. There are several driving forces for change, one being the recognition that unreasonable and unnecessary demands are often being made of students in the sheer volume of information which they are required to assimilate. This has prompted students, educators and health professionals alike to question, across the whole curriculum, the depth of knowledge which is required by the newly-qualified doctor and the means by which it should be achieved. The General Medical Council has recommended the development of a system-based core curriculum and has emphasised the crucial importance of integration between basic science and clinical medicine. These proposals have been welcomed and amplified, with respect to the teaching of neurology, by the Association of British Neurologists.

No area of medical science lends itself better than neuroscience to such a system-based, integrated approach and this has been the principal philosophy guiding the preparation of this book. Neuroscience, with all its sub-specialities both basic and clinical, is an enormous field where the growth of knowledge through research is exponential. This creates a great challenge to the medical educator in selecting what should comprise the core curriculum. It also signifies the potential for future advances in the diagnosis, prevention and treatment of neurological disease, recognised by the designation of the 1990s as the 'Decade of the Brain'.

Neuroanatomy is the cornerstone upon which is built an understanding of the nervous system and its disorders. The aim of this book, therefore, is to provide a clear and concise account of the anatomy of the human nervous system in sufficient detail to understand its main functions and the common disorders by which it is affected. An important feature of the book is the integration of neuroanatomy with illustrative clinical material. This has been done in order to show how a knowledge of neuroanatomy can help in the understanding of clinical symptoms and also to emphasise those areas of neuroanatomy which are particularly relevant to human neurological disease. We have introduced clinical concepts in the most elementary way to give a broad outline of the aetiology of nervous disease and the link with clinical diagnostic methods. Clinical material has been integrated as closely as possible with the relevant neuroanatomy. Furthermore, the clinical text has been boxed so that it is readily identifiable and can be easily selected to review or pass over. Each chapter also contains boxed summaries. The purpose of these is to assist the reader in identifying key points and as an aid to revision.

Both neuroanatomy and clinical medicine are new to the student first entering medical school. By studying the introductory chapter and the summaries of later, more detailed, chapters the student will gain an overview of the scope and extent of the subject of neuroanatomy and will be introduced to the basic concepts underlying the clinical diagnosis of neurological disease. For those unfamiliar with clinical terminology a glossary has been provided to explain the meaning of commonly used expressions. As more detailed knowledge of neuroanatomy is gained, this will be enhanced and illuminated by reference to the selected clinical material which exemplifies the relevance of neuroanatomy to clinical neurology. Later, when students enter neurological training, they need to refresh in their minds the basic principles of neuroanatomy and link these to clinical diagnostic methods. At this time, the systematic study of patients with individual neurological diseases can be greatly enhanced by returning to the detailed anatomy of diseased structures.

Manchester   **A R Crossman**
1995   **D Neary**

Acknowledgements

We wish to thank the numerous colleagues who have helped in many ways to bring this book to publication. At The University of Manchester, our thanks go to Raymond Evans, Denise Smith and Caroline Wilkinson, of the Unit of Art in Medicine, for their patient, imaginative and skilful transformation of our elementary sketches and verbal descriptions into the many drawings which illustrate this book. We are also grateful to the director of the unit, Richard Neave, for his interest in the project and for making himself so readily available with help and advice.

The book contains many photographs of anatomical specimens.

We are grateful to anatomical dissecting room technician John Davies for helping to select the most suitable anatomical specimens for prosection and to Tony Bentley for his meticulous photography. Specially for this new edition, many of the existing illustrations have been modified and improved and 18 entirely new figures have been added. We are particularly grateful to Ben Crossman for his work on figures 1.5, 1.11, 1.14, 1.20, 5.2, 5.3, 6.1(A), 6.1(B), 6.2, 6.3, 6.4, 6.5, 6.6, 6.9, 7.3, 8.6, 8.9(A), 8.9(B), 8.9(C), 8.9(D), 9.4, 9.5, 9.6, 9.7, 9.8, 9.9, 9.10, 9.11, 9.12, 9.13, 10.4, 10.8, 10.9, 10.11, 10.19, 11.1, 12.4, 13.22, 13.25, 14.2, 14.10, 16.7 and 16.10.

We are also indebted to Professor D J Brooks, Professor P D Griffiths, Professor A Jackson, Dr R A McKinney and Dr G C Schoenwolf for providing scans and other images.

The authors greatly appreciate the continued interest of the publishers in *Neuroanatomy* and the support and encouragement from colleagues at Elsevier Limited, particularly Publishing Manager Timothy Horne and Development Editor Helen Leng, in the preparation of this 3rd edition.

Manchester   A. R. C.
2004   D. N.

Contents

Chapter 1
Introduction and overview

The human nervous system is the most complex and versatile achievement of the process of evolution. The nervous system of all animals functions to detect changes in the external and internal environments and to bring about appropriate responses in muscles, organs and glands. With ascent of the evolutionary scale there is, in addition, an increasing capacity for 'higher functions' of the nervous system, such as learning, memory, cognition and, ultimately, self-awareness, intellect and personality. The anatomical, physiological, biochemical and molecular foundation of some aspects of neural function are well understood, while others continue to occupy the professional lives of many thousands of researchers in both the basic and clinical sciences.

The nervous system is often damaged by inherited or developmental abnormalities, by disease processes and by traumatic injury. The prevention, diagnosis and treatment of neurological disorders are, therefore, of immense socio-economic importance. An understanding of neuroanatomy and its correlation with function and dysfunction remains fundamental to the contemporary practice of clinical neuroscience and to the prospect of future advances.

Components and organisation of the nervous system

Neurones and neuroglia
The basic structural and functional unit of the nervous system is the nerve cell or **neurone** (Figs 1.1 and 1.2), of

which the human nervous system is estimated to contain about 10^{10}. The functions of the neurone are to receive and integrate incoming information from sensory receptors or other neurones and to transmit information to other neurones or effector organs. Neuronal structure is highly specialised to fulfil these functions. Each neurone is a separate entity with a limiting cell membrane. Information is passed between neurones at specialised regions called **synapses** where the membranes of adjacent cells are in close apposition (Fig. 1.1).

There is wide diversity in the shape and size of neurones in different parts of the nervous system, but all share certain common characteristics. There is a single cell body from which a variable number of branching processes emerge. Most of these processes are receptive in function and are known as **dendrites**. They possess synaptic specialisations,

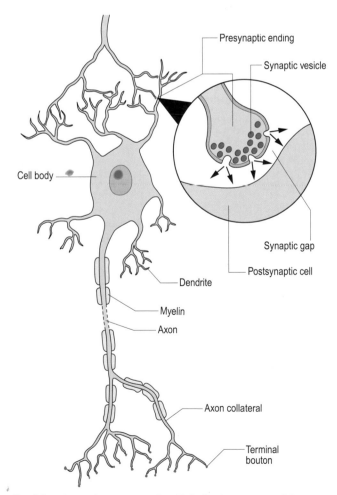

Fig. 1.1 **Schematic representation of the basic structure of the neurone and the synapse.**

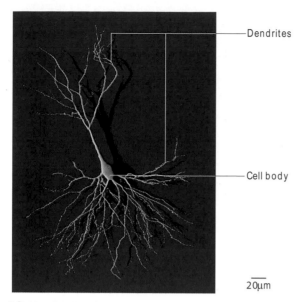

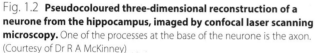

Fig. 1.2 **Pseudocoloured three-dimensional reconstruction of a neurone from the hippocampus, imaged by confocal laser scanning microscopy.** One of the processes at the base of the neurone is the axon. (Courtesy of Dr R A McKinney)

sometimes many thousands of them, through which they receive information from other nerve cells with which they make contact. In sensory neurones, the dendrites may be specialised to detect changes in the external or internal environment. One of the processes leaving the cell body is called the **axon** or nerve fibre and this carries information away from the cell body. Axons are highly variable in length and may divide into several branches or **collaterals** through which information can be distributed to a number of different destinations simultaneously. At the end of the axon, specialisations called **terminal boutons** occur; here information is transferred to the dendrites of other neurones.

Information is coded within neurones by changes in electrical energy. The neurone at rest possesses an electrical potential (the **resting potential**) across its membrane of the order of 60–70 millivolts, the inside being negative with respect to the outside. When a neurone is stimulated or excited above a certain threshold level, there is a brief reversal of the polarity of its membrane potential, termed the **action potential**. Action potentials are propagated down the axon and invade the nerve terminals. Transmission of information between neurones almost always occurs by chemical rather than electrical means. Invasion of nerve terminals by the action potential causes release of specific chemical agents that are stored in **synaptic vesicles** in the presynaptic ending. These chemicals are known as **neurotransmitters** and diffuse across the narrow gap between pre- and postsynaptic membranes to bind to **receptors** on the postsynaptic cell, inducing changes in the membrane potential. The change may be either to depolarise the membrane, thus moving towards the threshold for production of action potentials, or to hyperpolarise and, thus, stabilise the cell.

Neuroglial cells, or **glia**, constitute the other major cellular component of the nervous system, outnumbering neurones by an order of magnitude. Unlike neurones, neuroglia do not have a direct role in information processing but they fulfil a number of ancillary roles essential for the normal functioning of nerve cells. Three main types of neuroglial cell are recognised.

- **Oligodendrocytes** (oligodendroglia) form the **myelin sheath** that surrounds many neuronal axons (Fig. 1.1), conferring an increased rate of conduction of action potentials.
- **Astrocytes** are thought to form a selectively permeable barrier between the circulatory system and the neurones of the brain and spinal cord. This is known as the 'blood–brain barrier' and has a protective function.
- **Microglia** have a phagocytic role in the response to nervous system damage.

Central and peripheral nervous systems

The nervous system (Fig. 1.3) is divided arbitrarily into the **central nervous system (CNS)** and the **peripheral nervous system (PNS)**. The central nervous system consists of the brain and spinal cord, lying within the

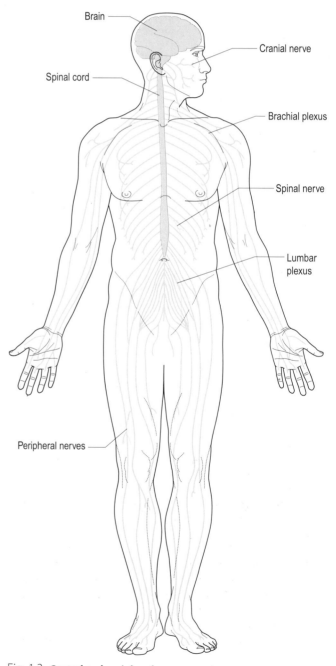

Fig. 1.3 **Central and peripheral nervous systems.**

protection of the cranium and vertebral column, respectively. This is the most complex part of the nervous system. It contains the majority of nerve cell bodies and synaptic connections. The peripheral nervous system constitutes the link between the CNS and structures in the periphery of the body, from which it receives sensory information and to which it sends controlling impulses. The peripheral nervous system consists of nerves joined to the brain and spinal cord (**cranial** and **spinal nerves**) and their ramifications within the body. Spinal nerves serving the upper or lower limbs coalesce to form the **brachial** or **lumbar plexus**, respectively, within which fibres are redistributed into named **peripheral nerves**. The PNS also encompasses some groups of peripherally located nerve cell bodies that are aggregated within structures called **ganglia**.

Autonomic nervous system

Neurones that detect changes in, and control the activity of, the viscera are collectively referred to as the autonomic nervous system. Its components are present in both the central and peripheral nervous systems. The autonomic nervous system is divided into two anatomically and functionally distinct parts, namely the **sympathetic** and **parasympathetic** divisions, which generally have antagonistic effects on the structures that they innervate. The autonomic nervous system innervates smooth muscle, cardiac muscle and secretory glands. It is an important part of the homeostatic mechanisms that control the internal environment of the body.

Afferent neurones, efferent neurones and interneurones

Nerve cells that carry information from peripheral receptors to the CNS are referred to as **afferent neurones** (Fig. 1.4). If the information that they carry ultimately reaches a conscious level they are also called **sensory neurones**. **Efferent neurones** carry impulses away from the CNS and if they innervate skeletal muscle to cause movement they are also referred to as **motor neurones**. The vast majority of neurones, however, reside entirely within the CNS and are usually called **interneurones** (the alternative terms

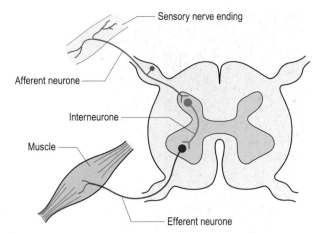

Fig. 1.4 **Examples of afferent, efferent and interneurones.**

internuncial and relay neurones are sometimes used). The terms 'afferent' and 'efferent' are also commonly used to denote the polarity of projections to and from structures within the CNS, even though the projections are entirely contained within the brain and spinal cord. The projections to and from the cerebral cortex, for example, are referred to as cortical afferents and efferents, respectively.

Grey and white matter, nuclei and tracts

The CNS is a highly heterogeneous structure in terms of the distribution of nerve cell bodies and their processes (Fig. 1.5). Some regions are relatively enriched in nerve cell bodies (e.g. the central portion of the spinal cord and the surface of the cerebral hemisphere) and are referred to as **grey matter**. Other regions contain mostly nerve processes (usually axons). These are often myelinated (ensheathed in myelin), which confers a paler coloration – hence the term **white matter**.

Nerve cell bodies with similar anatomical connections and functions (e.g. the motor neurones innervating a group of related muscles) tend to be located together in groups called **nuclei**. Similarly, nerve processes sharing common connections and functions tend to follow the same course, running in **pathways** or **tracts** (Figs 1.5 and 1.20).

Components and organisation of the nervous system

- The structural and functional unit of the nervous system is the nerve cell, or neurone. Neurones have a resting membrane potential of about –70 mV.
- A neurone receives information primarily through its dendrites and passes this on by action potentials, which are carried away from the cell body by the axon.
- Information is passed between neurones at synapses by release of neurotransmitter from presynaptic terminals; this acts upon receptors in the postsynaptic membrane to cause either depolarisation or hyperpolarisation of the postsynaptic cell.
- Neuroglial cells are more numerous than nerve cells but have ancillary roles and are not directly involved in information processing.
- Oligodendrocytes form the myelin sheath that surrounds axons and increases their rate of conduction.
- Astrocytes may form the blood–brain barrier.
- Microglia have a phagocytic function when the nervous system is damaged.

- The nervous system is divided into the central nervous system (CNS), which consists of the brain and spinal cord, and the peripheral nervous system, which consists of cranial and spinal nerves and their ramifications.
- The autonomic nervous system innervates visceral structures and is important in homeostasis of the internal environment.
- Individual neurones may be defined as either afferent or efferent with respect to the CNS, or as interneurones.
- Within the CNS, areas rich in either nerve cell bodies or nerve fibres constitute grey and white matter, respectively.
- Clusters of cell bodies with similar functions are known as nuclei.
- Tracts of nerve fibres link distant regions.
- Generally, ascending sensory and descending motor pathways in the CNS decussate along their course, so that each side of the brain is functionally associated with the contralateral half of the body.

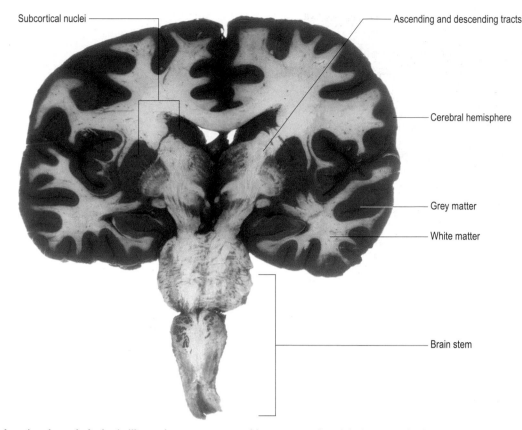

Fig. 1.5 **Coronal section through the brain illustrating grey matter, white matter and nuclei.** The section has been stained with Mulligan's stain which colours grey matter blue; white matter is relatively unstained.

Decussation of sensory and motor pathways

It is a general principle of the organisation of the CNS that pathways conveying sensory information to a conscious level (the cerebral hemisphere) cross over, or **decussate**, from one side of the CNS to the other. The same is true of descending pathways from the cerebral hemisphere that control movement. Therefore, in general, each cerebral hemisphere perceives sensations from, and controls the movements of, the contralateral side of the body.

Development of the central nervous system

By the beginning of the second week of human embryonic development, three germ cell layers become established: ectoderm, mesoderm and endoderm. Subsequently, these each give rise to particular tissues and organs in the adult. The ectoderm gives rise to the skin and the nervous system. The mesoderm forms skeletal, muscular and connective tissues. The endoderm gives rise to the alimentary, respiratory and genitourinary tracts. During the third week of embryonic development, the dorsal midline ectoderm undergoes thickening to form the **neural plate** (Figs 1.6 and 1.7). The lateral margins of the neural plate become elevated, forming **neural folds** on either side of a longitudinal, midline depression, the **neural groove**. The neural folds then become apposed and fuse together, thus sealing the neural groove and creating the **neural tube**. Some cells from the apices of the neural folds become separated to form groups lying dorsolateral to the neural tube. These are known as the **neural crests**. The formation of the neural tube is complete by about the middle of the fourth week of embryonic development.

Enormous growth, distortion and cellular differentiation occur during the subsequent transformation of the neural tube into the adult CNS. This is maximal in the rostral part, which develops into the brain, the caudal portion becoming the spinal cord. The central cavity within the neural tube becomes the central canal of the spinal cord and the ventricles of the brain. The neural crests form the sensory ganglia of spinal and cranial nerves, and also the autonomic ganglia.

As development continues, a longitudinal groove, the **sulcus limitans**, appears on the inner surface of the lateral walls of the embryonic spinal cord and caudal part of the brain (Fig. 1.8A). The dorsal and ventral cell groupings thus delineated are referred to as the **alar plate** and the **basal plate**, respectively. Nerve cells that develop within the alar plate have predominantly sensory functions, while those in the basal plate are predominantly motor. Further development also brings about the differentiation of grey and white matter. The grey matter is located centrally around the central canal, with white matter forming an outer coat. This basic developmental pattern can still easily be recognised in the adult spinal cord (Fig. 1.8B).

During embryonic development, the rostral portion of the neural tube undergoes massive differentiation and growth to form the brain (Fig. 1.9). By about the fifth week, three primary brain vesicles can be identified: the **prosencephalon** (forebrain), **mesencephalon** (midbrain) and **rhombencephalon** (hindbrain). The longitudinal axis of the developing CNS (neuraxis) does not remain straight but is bent by a midbrain or cephalic flexure, occurring at the junction of midbrain and forebrain, and a cervical flexure between the brain and the spinal cord.

By the seventh week further differentiation distinguishes five secondary brain vesicles produced by division of the

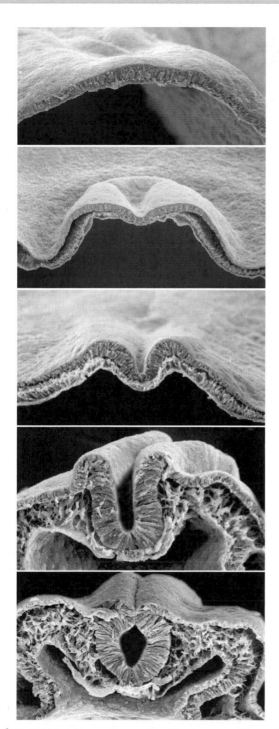

Fig. 1.6 **Scanning electron micrographs of transverse sections through the dorsal ectoderm of the chick embryo illustrating the stages (from top to bottom) in formation of the neural tube (×140).** (Courtesy of Dr G C Schoenwolf)

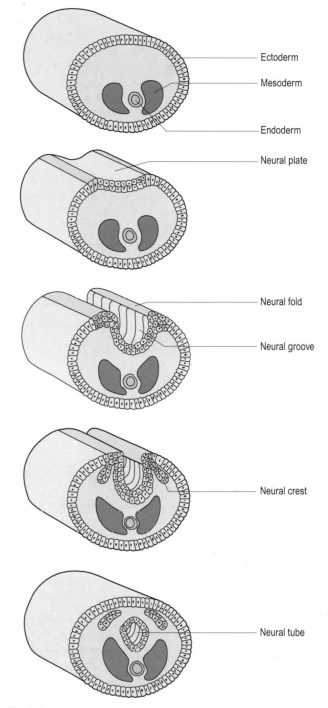

Fig. 1.7 **Schematic representation of the formation of the neural tube from the embryonic ectoderm.**

Table 1.1	**Embryonic development of the brain**	
Primary brain vesicles	**Secondary brain vesicles**	**Derivatives in mature brain**
Prosencephalon (forebrain)	Telencephalon	Cerebral hemisphere
	Diencephalon	Thalamus
Mesencephalon (midbrain)	Mesencephalon	Midbrain
Rhombencephalon (hindbrain)	Metencephalon	Pons, cerebellum
	Myelencephalon	Medulla oblongata

prosencephalon into the **telencephalon** and **diencephalon** and division of the rhombencephalon into the **metencephalon** and **myelencephalon**. The junction between the latter is marked by an additional bend in the neuraxis, called the pontine flexure.

Some of the names of the embryological subdivisions of the brain are commonly used for descriptive purposes and it is, therefore, useful to know the parts of the mature brain into which they subsequently develop (Table 1.1). Of the three basic divisions of the brain, the prosencephalon or forebrain is by far the largest. It is also referred to as the **cerebrum**. Within the cerebrum, the telencephalon undergoes the greatest further development and gives rise to

the two **cerebral hemispheres**. These consist of an outer layer of grey matter (the **cerebral cortex**) and an inner mass of white matter, within which various groups of nuclei lie buried (the largest being the **corpus striatum**). The diencephalon consists largely of the **thalamus**, which

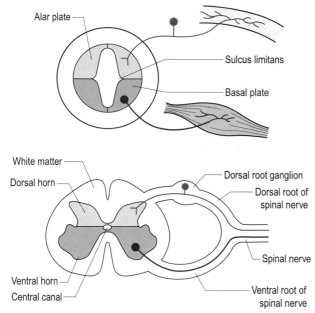

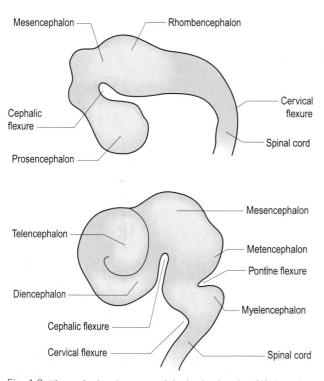

Fig. 1.8 **Schematic representation of transverse sections through (A) the developing neural tube and (B) the adult spinal cord.** Neuronal connections with peripheral structures are only illustrated on one side.

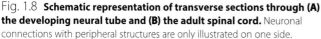

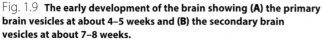

Fig. 1.9 **The early development of the brain showing (A) the primary brain vesicles at about 4–5 weeks and (B) the secondary brain vesicles at about 7–8 weeks.**

contains numerous cell groupings and is intimately connected with the cerebral cortex. The mesencephalon, or midbrain, is relatively undifferentiated (it still retains a central tube-like cavity surrounded by grey matter). The metencephalon develops into the **pons** and overlying **cerebellum**, while the myelencephalon forms the **medulla oblongata** (medulla). By convention, the medulla, pons and midbrain are collectively referred to as the **brain stem** (Fig. 1.10).

As the brain develops, its central cavity also undergoes considerable changes in size and shape, forming a system of

chambers or **ventricles** (Figs 1.10 and 1.19) which contain **cerebrospinal fluid** (CSF).

Parallels have been drawn between the embryological development of the brain and the major changes that the brain has undergone during ascent of the phylogenetic, or evolutionary, scale from simple to more complex animals. While this is certainly an oversimplification, the concept does have the advantage of introducing some of the principal parts of the brain, and their relationships to one another, in a graphic and memorable way (Fig. 1.10).

The simplest of chordate animals (e.g. amphioxus), from which the vertebrates evolved, possesses a dorsal tubular nerve cord that is reminiscent of the neural tube of the developing mammalian embryo. During phylogeny, the rostral end of the tubular nervous system has undergone enormous modification and change; consequently, the adult human brain bears little obvious similarity to its evolutionary ancestors.

Regional specialisation has been an important theme in the evolution of the brain and this is especially obvious in relation to the senses and in movement control. Long ago in phylogeny, centres devoted to these functions developed as expansions or outgrowths from the dorsal aspect of the simple tubular brain (Fig. 1.10). In form, they consisted of an outer cortex of nerve cell bodies with an underlying core of nerve fibres. Bilaterally paired centres developed in relation to the senses of smell, vision and hearing, and a symmetrical, midline centre developed in association with vestibular function and the maintenance of equilibrium. Each of these centres underwent subsequent evolutionary change, but this was most evident in the rostral, 'olfactory', part of the brain, which developed into the massive cerebral hemispheres (Figs 1.11 and 1.12). During this process of prosencephalisation, the cerebral hemispheres came to take on an executive role in many areas of brain function. For example, the highest level for perception and correlation of all sensory modalities eventually became localised in the cortical surface of the cerebral hemispheres, as did the highest level for motor control. This is reflected by the fact that only a small proportion of the adult human cerebral hemisphere remains directly related to olfactory function.

The process of prosencephalisation meant that the other centres became progressively subservient to the cerebral hemispheres. For example, those for vision and hearing underwent relatively little development and fulfil largely automatic, reflex functions in the human brain. They may

> ### Developmental anomalies
> Disorders of development disrupt the normal growth and structural organisation of the spinal cord and brain. Because the nervous system is derived from embryonic ectoderm, these developmental anomalies also involve the coverings of the nervous system (skin and bone). In **anencephaly**, the brain and skull are minute and the infant does not usually survive. In **spina bifida**, the lower spinal cord and nerve roots are underdeveloped and may lie uncovered by skin or the bony spine on the infant's back (**meningiomyelocele**). Such infants are left with withered, paralysed and anaesthetic lower limbs together with incontinence of the bowel and bladder.

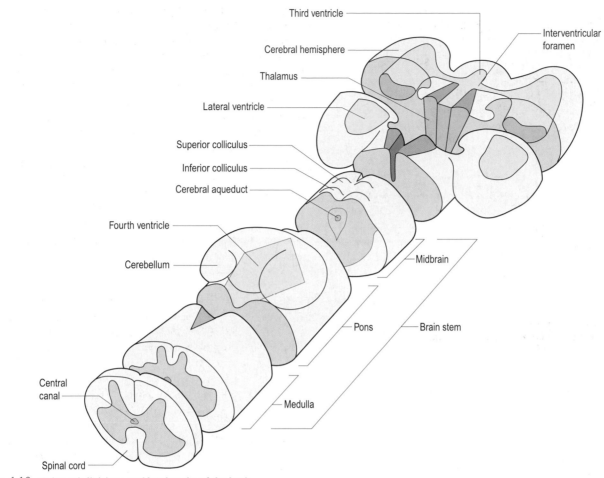

Fig. 1.10 **Major subdivisions and landmarks of the brain.**

still be identified, however, as four small swellings on the dorsal surface of the midbrain: the **corpora quadrigemina** or **superior** and **inferior colliculi** (Figs 1.10–1.12). The motor centre near the caudal end of the brain developed into the cerebellum (Figs 1.10–1.12), which retains a central role in the maintenance of equilibrium and the coordination of movement.

Overview of the anatomy of the central nervous system

Coverings and blood supply

The brain and spinal cord are supported and protected by the bones of the skull and vertebral column. Within these bony coverings the CNS is entirely ensheathed by three layers of membranes, called the **meninges** (Fig. 1.13). The outermost membrane is the **dura mater**, a tough, fibrous coat that surrounds the brain and spinal cord like a loose-fitting bag. The spinal dura and much of the cranial dura are separate from the periosteum, which lines the surrounding bones. At certain locations, however, such as the floor of the cranial cavity, the dura and periosteum are fused and the cranial dura is tightly adherent to the interior of the skull. Two large sheets of dura project into the cranial cavity, incompletely dividing it into compartments (Fig. 1.14). The **falx cerebri** lies in the sagittal plane between the two cerebral hemispheres. Its free border lies above the corpus callosum. The **tentorium cerebelli** is oriented horizontally, lying beneath the occipital lobes of the cerebral hemispheres

and above the cerebellum. The dura mater can be regarded as consisting of two layers. These are fused together except in certain locations where they become separated to form spaces, the **dural venous sinuses**, which serve as channels for the venous drainage of the brain. Important dural sinuses occur:

- on the floor of the cranial cavity
- along the lines of attachment of the falx cerebri and tentorium cerebelli to the interior of the skull (superior sagittal sinus, Fig. 1.14; transverse sinus)

> ### Coverings and blood supply of the central nervous system
>
> - The brain and spinal cord are invested by three meningeal layers: the dura mater, arachnoid mater and pia mater.
> - Two sheets of cranial dura mater, the falx cerebri and tentorium cerebelli, incompletely divide the cranial cavity into compartments.
> - The cranial dura mater contains dural venous sinuses, which act as channels for the venous drainage of the brain.
> - Beneath the arachnoid mater lies the subarachnoid space in which CSF circulates.
> - The brain is supplied with blood by the internal carotid and vertebral arteries.
> - The spinal cord is supplied by vessels arising from the vertebral arteries, reinforced by radicular arteries derived from segmental vessels.

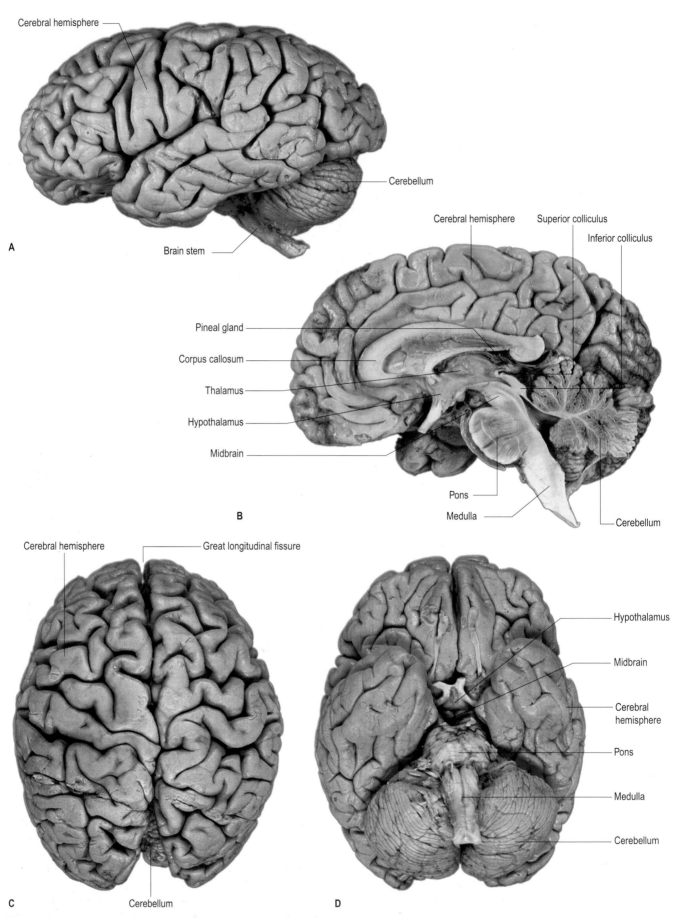

Fig. 1.11 **Photographs of the brain.** (**A**) Lateral aspect; (**B**) median sagittal section; (**C**) dorsal aspect; (**D**) ventral aspect.

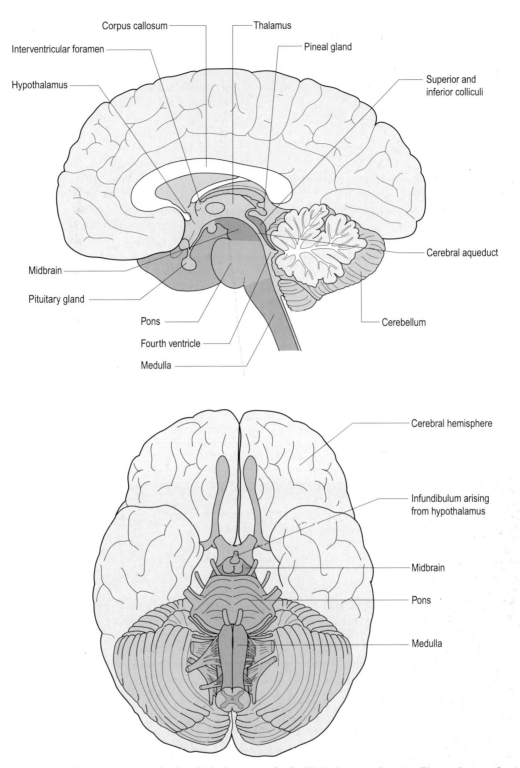

Corpus callosum
Interventricular foramen
Hypothalamus
Thalamus
Pineal gland
Superior and inferior colliculi
Cerebral aqueduct
Midbrain
Pituitary gland
Cerebellum
Pons
Fourth ventricle
Medulla

A

Cerebral hemisphere
Infundibulum arising from hypothalamus
Midbrain
Pons
Medulla

B

Fig. 1.12 **Principal subdivisions and some important landmarks in the mature brain.** (**A**) Median sagittal section; (**B**) ventral aspect. Cranial nerves are indicated in yellow.

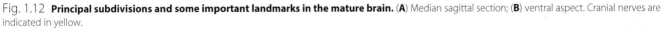

■ along the line of attachment of the falx cerebri and tentorium cerebelli to one another (straight sinus).

Beneath the dura lies the **arachnoid mater**, the two being separated by a thin **subdural space**. The arachnoid is a translucent, collagenous membrane that, like the dura, loosely envelops the brain and spinal cord. The innermost of the meninges is the **pia mater**, a delicate membrane of microscopic thickness that is firmly adherent to the surface of the brain and spinal cord, closely following their contours. Between the arachnoid and pia is the **subarachnoid space** through which CSF circulates.

The brain is supplied with arterial blood by the **internal carotid** and **vertebral arteries**, which anastomose to form the **circle of Willis** (circulus arteriosus) on the base of the brain. The spinal cord is supplied by vessels arising from the vertebral arteries, reinforced by **radicular arteries** derived from segmental vessels. The arteries and veins serving the CNS run for part of their course within the subarachnoid space (Fig. 1.13). The meninges are supplied by a number of vessels, the most significant intracranial one being the **middle meningeal artery**, which ramifies extensively between the skull and dura mater overlying the lateral aspect of the cerebral hemisphere.

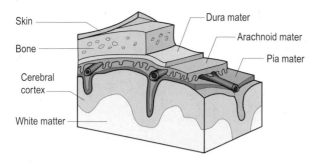

Fig. 1.13 **A section through the skull, illustrating the relationships between the meninges and the CNS.**

Anatomy of the spinal cord

The spinal cord lies within the **vertebral (spinal) canal** of the vertebral column and is continuous rostrally with the medulla oblongata of the brain stem (Fig. 1.15). The spinal cord receives information from, and controls, the trunk and limbs. This is achieved through 31 pairs of **spinal nerves**, which join the cord at intervals along its length and contain afferent and efferent nerve fibres connecting with structures in the periphery. Near to the cord, the spinal nerves divide into **dorsal** and **ventral roots**, which attach to the cord along its dorsolateral and ventrolateral borders, respectively (Fig. 1.16). The dorsal roots carry afferent fibres, the cell bodies of which are located in **dorsal root ganglia**. The ventral roots carry efferent fibres with cell bodies lying

within the spinal grey matter. Spinal nerves leave the vertebral canal through small holes, called **intervertebral foramina**, between adjacent vertebrae (Fig. 1.17). Because of a difference in the rates of growth of the spinal cord and vertebral column during development, the spinal cord in the adult does not extend the full length of the vertebral canal but ends at the level of the intervertebral disc between L1 and L2. The lumbar and sacral spinal nerves, therefore, descend in a leash-like arrangement, the **cauda equina** (Fig. 1.15), to reach their exit point.

The spinal cord is a relatively undifferentiated structure compared with the brain. Consequently, the basic principles of organisation, established early in embryonic development, can be readily identified even in the adult human cord (Fig. 1.16). The spinal cord is approximately cylindrical in shape, containing at its centre a vestigial **central canal**. The separation of cell bodies from nerve fibres gives a characteristic 'H' or 'butterfly' shape to the central core of grey matter that surrounds the central canal. Four extensions of the central grey matter project dorsolaterally and ventrolaterally towards the lines of attachment of the dorsal and ventral roots of the spinal nerves. These are known as **dorsal horns** and **ventral horns**, respectively. The dorsal horn is the site of termination of many afferent neurones conveying impulses from sensory receptors throughout the body and is the site of origin of ascending pathways carrying sensory impulses to the brain. The ventral horn contains motor neurones that innervate skeletal muscle. In addition,

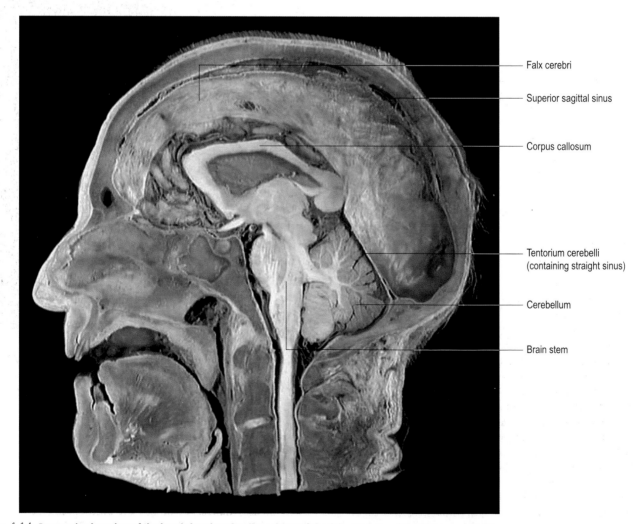

Fig. 1.14 **Parasagittal section of the head showing the disposition of the falx cerebri and tentorium cerebelli.**

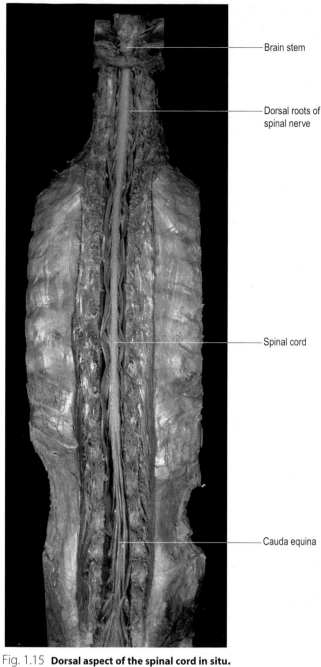

Fig. 1.15 **Dorsal aspect of the spinal cord in situ.**

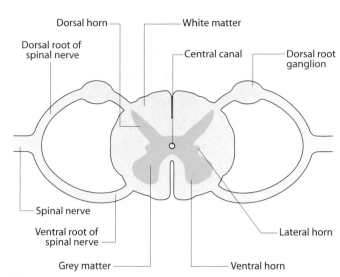

Fig. 1.16 **Schematic diagram of a transverse section through the spinal cord, showing the attachment of spinal nerve roots and the arrangement of grey and white matter.**

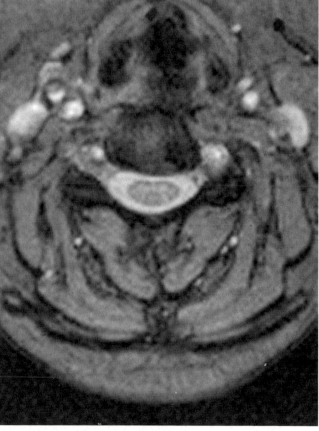

Fig. 1.17 **Transaxial (transverse) magnetic resonance image of the spine.** (Courtesy of Professor A Jackson)

Anatomy of the spinal cord

- The spinal cord lies within the vertebral canal and bears 31 pairs of spinal nerves through which it receives fibres from and sends fibres to the periphery.
- Near the cord, spinal nerves divide to form dorsal and ventral roots; dorsal roots carry afferent fibres with cell bodies in dorsal root ganglia, and ventral roots carry efferent fibres.
- The spinal cord consists of a central core of grey matter, containing nerve cell bodies, and an outer layer of white matter or nerve fibres.
- Within the grey matter, the dorsal horn contains sensory neurones, the ventral horn contains motor neurones and the lateral horn contains preganglionic sympathetic neurones.
- Within the white matter run ascending and descending nerve fibre tracts, which link the spinal cord with the brain.
- The principal ascending tracts are the dorsal columns, the spinothalamic tracts and the spinocerebellar tracts. The corticospinal tract is an important descending tract.

at thoracic and upper lumbar levels of the cord only, another, smaller, collection of cell bodies comprises the **lateral horn**, which contains preganglionic neurones belonging to the sympathetic division of the autonomic nervous system.

The periphery of the cord consists of white matter that contains longitudinally running nerve fibres. These are organised into a series of ascending tracts, which carry

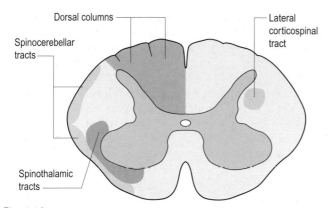

Fig. 1.18 **Diagram of a transverse section through the spinal cord showing the locations of the principal ascending (left side) and descending (right side) nerve fibre tracts.**

information from the trunk and limbs to the brain, and descending tracts, by which the brain controls the activities of neurones in the spinal cord (Fig. 1.18). The principal ascending tracts are the **dorsal columns** (fasciculus gracilis and fasciculus cuneatus), which carry fine touch and proprioception, the **spinothalamic tracts**, which carry pain, temperature, coarse touch and pressure, and the **spinocerebellar tracts**, which carry information from muscle and joint receptors to the cerebellum. Amongst the descending tracts, one of the most important is the **lateral corticospinal tract**, which controls skilled voluntary movements.

Anatomy of the brain

Major features and landmarks
The brain is dominated by the massive **cerebral hemispheres** (Figs 1.11 and 1.12). These have a highly convoluted outer mantle of grey matter and an inner core of white matter. Certain of the surface convolutions subserve specific sensory or motor functions, described below. The two cerebral hemispheres are incompletely separated by the **great longitudinal fissure**. The fissure is normally occupied by the falx cerebri and in its depths lies the **corpus callosum**, containing commissural fibres that unite corresponding regions of the two hemispheres.

The **brain stem** can be seen clearly when the brain is viewed ventrally, although the relationships of the midbrain are best illustrated in sagittal section. The brain stem is the origin of **cranial nerves** III–XII. Dorsal (posterior) to the brain stem is located the cerebellum. The tentorium cerebelli normally lies between the cerebellum and the posterior part (occipital lobes) of the cerebral hemispheres.

Ventricular system
The highly simplified plan of the basic brain, described above, is a useful one on which to consider the general disposition of the ventricular system (Figs 1.10, 1.12 and 1.19). As the central canal of the spinal cord ascends into the brain stem it moves progressively in a dorsal direction, eventually opening out to form a shallow, rhomboid-shaped depression on the dorsal surface of the medulla and pons (the hindbrain portion of the brain stem) beneath the cerebellum. This is the **fourth ventricle**.

At the rostral border of the pons, the walls of the fourth ventricle converge, forming once again a narrow tube, the **cerebral aqueduct** (Figs 1.10, 1.12 and 1.19). The cerebral aqueduct dives into the substance of the brain stem running the length of the midbrain beneath the inferior and superior colliculi. At the junction of midbrain and forebrain, the aqueduct opens into the **third ventricle** (Figs 1.10, 1.12 and 1.19), a slit-like chamber, narrow from side to side but extensive in dorsoventral and rostrocaudal dimensions. The lateral walls of the third ventricle are formed by the thalamus and hypothalamus of the diencephalon. Near the rostral end of the third ventricle a small aperture, the **interventricular foramen** or **foramen of Monro**

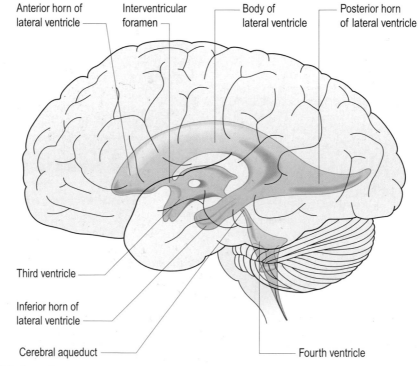

Fig. 1.19 **The cerebral ventricular system.**

(Figs 1.10, 1.12 and 1.19), communicates with an extensive chamber, the **lateral ventricle** (Figs 1.10 and 1.19), within each cerebral hemisphere. The ventricular system is the site of production of CSF, which is secreted by the **choroid plexus**.

Brain stem

When the brain is viewed externally, the massive cerebral hemispheres obscure many other structures, but a median sagittal section (Figs 1.11B and 1.12A) reveals most of the main features of the basic brain. The brain stem can be clearly seen on both a median sagittal section and a ventral view (Figs 1.11 and 1.12) of the brain. The brain stem consists of the medulla oblongata, pons and midbrain, each of which can be readily delineated.

The brain stem forms only a small proportion of the entire brain but it is crucially important. Through it pass ascending and descending nerve fibre tracts linking the brain and spinal cord (Fig. 1.20). These carry sensory information from, and permit movement of, the trunk and limbs. The brain stem also contains the sites of origin and termination of many of the **cranial nerves** through which the brain innervates the head region. Moreover, within the brain stem lie centres controlling vital functions such as respiration, the cardiovascular system and the level of consciousness.

The medulla oblongata is continuous caudally with the spinal cord and extends rostrally as far as the pons. The latter junction can clearly be seen on ventral or sagittal views since the ventral part of the pons forms a prominent bulge on the surface of the brain stem. In sagittal section (Figs 1.11B and 1.12A), the lumen of the fourth ventricle is apparent between the pons and medulla ventrally and the cerebellum dorsally, into which its tent-shaped roof extends.

Cranial nerves

The brain receives sensory information from, and controls the activities of, peripheral structures, principally the head and neck. Afferent and efferent nerve fibres run in 12 pairs of cranial nerves, which are identified by individual names and Roman numerals I–XII. Certain of the cranial nerves contain only sensory or motor nerve fibres but the majority, like spinal nerves, contain a mixture. The first two cranial nerves (I olfactory, II optic) attach directly to the forebrain and the rest attach to the brain stem. Within the brain stem lie a number of cell groupings, called the **cranial nerve nuclei**. These are the sites of termination of sensory fibres and the origin of the motor fibres (Fig. 1.20) that run in the cranial nerves.

Cerebellum

The cerebellum is attached to the brain stem by a large mass of nerve fibres that lie lateral to the fourth ventricle on either side. It is split nominally into three parts: the **inferior, middle** and **superior cerebellar peduncles**.

These carry nerve fibres between the medulla, pons and midbrain, respectively, and the cerebellum. The largest cerebellar peduncle is the middle and it is the only one readily seen without further dissection (Fig. 1.12B). The cerebellum consists of an outer layer of grey matter, the cerebellar cortex, surrounding a central core of white matter. The cortical surface is highly convoluted to form a regular pattern of narrow, parallel folds or **folia**. The cerebellar white matter consists of nerve fibres running to and from the cerebellar cortex. The white matter has a characteristic branching, tree-like arrangement in section (Fig. 1.11; see also Fig. 8.8), as its ramifications reach towards the surface. The cerebellum is concerned with the coordination of movement and operates at an entirely unconscious level.

Rostral to the pons is located the relatively small midbrain. On its dorsal surface can be seen the rounded eminences of the superior and inferior colliculi, beneath which runs the cerebral aqueduct (Figs 1.10–1.12).

Diencephalon and cerebral hemispheres

Rostral to the brain stem lies the forebrain, consisting of the diencephalon and cerebral hemispheres. The diencephalon

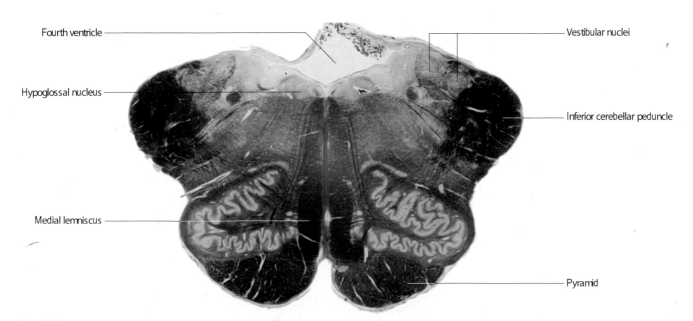

Fig. 1.20 **Transverse section through the brain stem at the level of the medulla oblongata.** The section has been stained by the Weigert–Pal method. Areas rich in nerve fibres stain darkly while areas rich in cell bodies are relatively paler. The pyramid contains descending motor fibres which run from the cerebral cortex to the spinal cord. The medial lemniscus consists of ascending axons carrying sensory information from the limbs to higher centres in the brain. The inferior cerebellar peduncle contains spinocerebellar fibres carrying information from joints and muscles to the cerebellum. The vestibular nuclei are the site of termination of the vestibular nerve. The hypoglossal nucleus is the site of origin of hypoglossal nerve fibres.

and cerebral hemisphere on each side of the brain are to a large extent physically separate from their counterparts on the other side, although important cross-connections do exist, as described below. The two sides of the diencephalon are separated by the lumen of the third ventricle, whose lateral walls they constitute.

The diencephalon consists of four main subdivisions in a dorsoventral direction: the **epithalamus**, **thalamus**, **subthalamus** and **hypothalamus**. The epithalamus is small and its most notable component on a sagittal section is the **pineal gland**, which lies in the midline immediately rostral to the superior colliculi of the midbrain (Fig. 1.12A). The thalamus is by far the largest part of the diencephalon and it forms much of the lateral wall of the third ventricle. The thalamus plays an important part in sensory, motor and cognitive functions and has extensive connections with the cerebral cortex. Little of the subthalamus can be seen and its structure and function are considered elsewhere (Chapter 12). The hypothalamus forms the lower part of the walls and floor of the third ventricle. It is a highly complex and important region because of its involvement in many systems, most notably the autonomic nervous system (Chapter 4), the limbic system and the neuro-endocrine system (Chapter 16). From the ventral aspect of the hypothalamus in the midline arises the **infundibulum** or pituitary stalk, to which is attached the **pituitary gland** (Fig. 1.12).

The cerebral hemisphere is by far the largest part of the brain. Like the cerebellum, it consists of an outer layer, or cortex, of grey matter and an inner mass of white matter (Figs 1.21 and 1.22). In addition, partly buried within the white matter lie several large subcortical masses of cell bodies collectively referred to as the **basal ganglia** (Figs 1.5, 1.21 and 1.22). The two cerebral hemispheres are separated by a deep midline cleft, the **great longitudinal fissure** (Fig. 1.21), which accommodates the **falx cerebri**, a sheet of dura mater reflected from the internal surface of the cranium. In the depths of the fissure lies the **corpus callosum** (Figs 1.12A and 1.21), a large sheet of transversely running nerve fibres (commissural fibres) that link corresponding areas of the two cerebral cortices.

The cerebral cortex is highly convoluted. This has the effect of maximising the cortical surface area, which is over 1 m² for each hemisphere. The convolutions are called **gyri** (singular: gyrus) and the furrows between them are **sulci** (singular: sulcus). Some gyri and sulci have a relatively consistent configuration between individuals and they mark the location of important functional areas.

On the lateral surface of the hemisphere, a deep cleft, the **lateral fissure** (Figs 1.21 and 1.23), is an important landmark. This, together with certain sulci, forms boundaries that divide the hemisphere into four lobes (Figs 1.23 and 1.24). The lobes bear the names of the bones of the skull beneath which they lie.

The most anterior part of the cerebral hemisphere is called the **frontal lobe**, the most anterior convexity of which is the frontal pole. The posterior boundary of the frontal lobe is the **central sulcus**, which can be identified as a single, continuous furrow running over the entire lateral surface of the hemisphere from the great longitudinal fissure to the lateral fissure. Posterior to the central sulcus lies the **parietal lobe**, which is separated from the **temporal lobe** below by the lateral fissure. The tip of the temporal lobe is called the temporal pole. The posterior part of the hemisphere is the **occipital lobe**, ending in the occipital pole. The boundaries between parietal and temporal lobes and the occipital lobe are indistinct on the lateral surface of the hemisphere since they do not correspond to any particular sulci; however, on the medial surface parietal and occipital lobes are separated by a deep **parieto-occipital sulcus** (Fig. 1.24).

The functions of the cerebral cortex are described in more detail in Chapter 13. It will be useful at the outset, however,

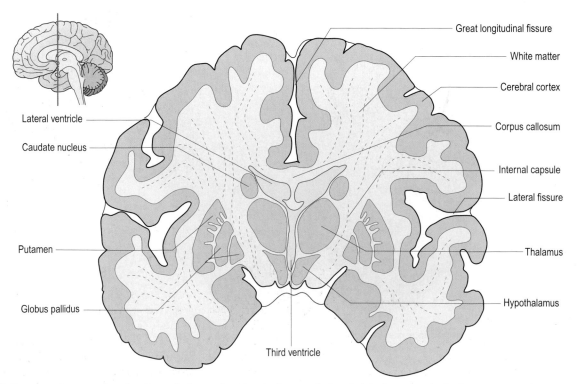

Great longitudinal fissure

White matter

Cerebral cortex

Corpus callosum

Internal capsule

Lateral fissure

Thalamus

Hypothalamus

Lateral ventricle

Caudate nucleus

Putamen

Globus pallidus

Third ventricle

Fig. 1.21 **Drawing of a coronal section through the cerebral hemisphere at the level of the interventricular foramen.**

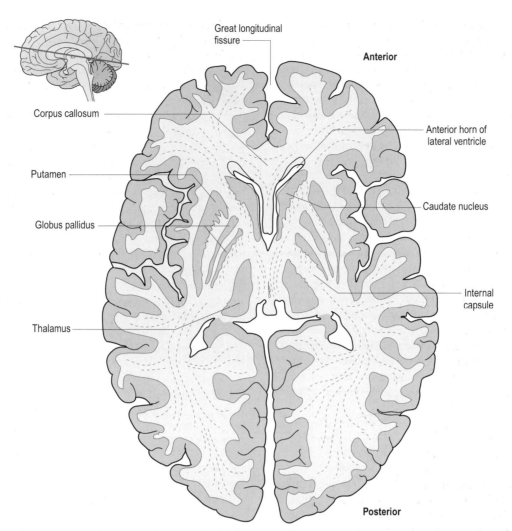

Fig. 1.22 **Drawing of an approximately horizontal section through the cerebral hemisphere.**

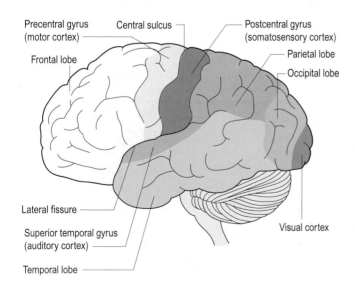

Fig. 1.23 **Lateral aspect of the brain.** The figure illustrates some of the principal gyri, sulci and functional areas.

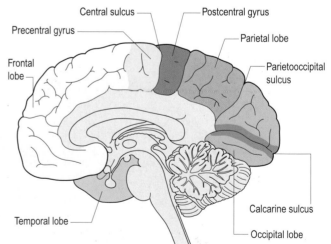

Fig. 1.24 **Sagittal section of the brain.** The figure illustrates some of the principal gyri, sulci and functional areas.

to identify four important functional areas of cortex, one in each lobe (Figs 1.23 and 1.24).

- In the frontal lobe, the gyrus immediately in front of the central sulcus is referred to anatomically as the **precentral gyrus**. Functionally, this contains the **primary motor cortex**, which is the highest level in the

brain for the control of movement. Here, in each hemisphere, the opposite half of the body is represented in a highly precise fashion.

- In the parietal lobe, facing the primary motor cortex across the central sulcus, lies the **postcentral gyrus** or **primary somatosensory cortex**. This is the site of termination of pathways carrying the modalities of touch, pressure, pain and temperature from the opposite half of the body and it is the region where they are consciously perceived. The special senses have their highest level of representation in other areas.

■ The **visual cortex** is located in the occipital lobe, mostly on the medial aspect of the hemisphere in the gyri above and below the horizontally orientated **calcarine sulcus**.

■ In the temporal lobe lies the **auditory cortex**. It is localised to the **superior temporal gyrus**, which lies beneath, and parallel to, the lateral fissure.

During development, the cerebral hemisphere takes on a C-shaped configuration as a result of the forward migration of the temporal lobe, such that the temporal pole lies adjacent to the frontal lobe and separated from it by the lateral fissure. The lateral ventricle within the hemisphere, therefore, is also basically C-shaped with 'horns' extending into the frontal, occipital and temporal lobes (Fig. 1.19).

The basic structure of the cerebral hemisphere is an outer mantle of grey matter, the cerebral cortex, beneath which lies a large and complex mass of white matter consisting of nerve fibres running to and from the cortex (Figs 1.21, 1.22 and 1.25).

Cortical afferent and efferent fibres which pass between the cerebral cortex and subcortical structures such as the corpus striatum, thalamus, brain stem and spinal cord are arranged in a characteristic radiating pattern, the **corona radiata**, which reaches out to the convolutions of the cortical surface (Fig. 1.25). Deeper inside the hemisphere the fibres are concentrated into a dense sheet of white matter, known as the **internal capsule** (Figs 1.21, 1.22 and 1.25).

Deep inside the hemisphere, both medial and lateral to the internal capsule, lie additional masses of grey matter, often collectively referred to as the **basal ganglia**. The largest of these is the **corpus striatum**, which consists of the **caudate nucleus, putamen** and **globus pallidus** (Figs 1.21 and 1.22). The caudate nucleus lies in the wall of

---

Basic organisation of the brain

■ The brain is conventionally divided into hindbrain, midbrain and forebrain.
■ The hindbrain is further subdivided into the medulla oblongata, pons and cerebellum.
■ The medulla, pons and midbrain constitute the brain stem.
■ The forebrain consists of the diencephalon (thalamus and hypothalamus) and the cerebral hemisphere.
■ Within the cerebral hemisphere lie several large nuclei called the basal ganglia or corpus striatum.
■ The brain contains a system of cavities or ventricles containing CSF, which is produced by the choroid plexus.
■ The brain possesses 12 pairs of cranial nerves, which carry afferent and efferent fibres.
■ The two cerebral hemispheres are linked by the fibres of the corpus callosum.
■ The surface of the cerebral hemisphere consists of cortical grey matter, which is folded to form gyri and sulci. Beneath the surface lie the dense fibre masses of the corona radiata and the internal capsule. The surface is divided into four lobes:
— frontal lobe containing the primary motor and premotor cortices
— parietal lobe containing the primary somatosensory cortex
— temporal lobe containing the primary auditory cortex
— occipital lobe containing the primary visual cortex.

---

the lateral ventricle throughout its extent and, like the ventricle, it is C-shaped. The basal ganglia are concerned with the control of muscle tone, posture and movement.

The major sensory pathways

Sensory information about the internal and external environment is carried to the CNS in afferent nerve fibres

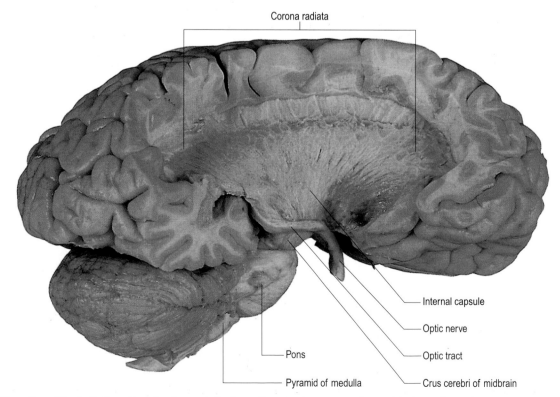

Fig. 1.25 **Dissection of the brain from the lateral aspect.** The figure illustrates the corona radiata and the internal capsule.

running in cranial and spinal nerves. Sensory information can be classified under the headings of 'special senses' and 'general senses'. The special senses are all carried in cranial nerves and comprise olfaction (I), vision (II), taste (VII and IX), and hearing and vestibular function (VIII). The special senses are dealt with in more detail elsewhere.

The general senses include the modalities of touch, pressure, pain and temperature (relayed from exteroceptors in the skin and interoceptors in the viscera), and awareness of posture and movement (from proprioceptors in joints, tendons and muscles). General sensory information from the trunk and limbs is carried in spinal nerves; from the head it is carried in the trigeminal nerve (cranial nerve V).

For all modalities in the category of general sensation, there is a sequence of three neurones between the sensory receptor located in the periphery and the perception of sensation at the level of the cerebral cortex (Fig. 1.26). The first neurone (first-order neurone or primary afferent neurone) enters the spinal cord, or the brain stem, through a spinal nerve, or the trigeminal nerve, on the same side of the body as its peripheral receptor is located. The cell body of the first-order neurone is located in the dorsal root ganglion of a spinal nerve, or in the trigeminal ganglion. Within the CNS, the first-order neurone remains ipsilateral and synapses upon the second neurone (second-order neurone), the exact location of its termination depending on the modality concerned. The second neurone has its cell body in the spinal cord or brain stem. Its axon crosses over (decussates) to the other side of the CNS and ascends to the thalamus, where it terminates. The third neurone in the sequence has its cell body in the thalamus and its axon projects to the somatosensory cortex, located in the parietal lobe of the cerebral hemisphere.

More specifically, primary spinal afferents carrying coarse touch/pressure, pain and temperature information terminate near their level of entry into the cord. They synapse with second-order neurones, the axons of which decussate within a few segments and thereafter form the spinothalamic tract. Primary spinal afferents carrying proprioceptive information and discriminative (fine) touch ascend uninterrupted on the same side of the cord, forming the dorsal columns (fasciculus gracilis and fasciculus cuneatus). They terminate in the dorsal column nuclei (nuclei gracilis and cuneatus) located in the medulla. From here, second-order neurones decussate and ascend to the thalamus as the medial lemniscus. Primary afferent neurones that enter the brain stem in the trigeminal nerve terminate ipsilaterally in the trigeminal sensory nucleus, one of the cranial nerve nuclei. From here, second-order neurones decussate and ascend to the thalamus as the trigeminothalamic tract. Second-order sensory neurones, of either spinal cord or brain-stem origin, converge upon the same region of the thalamus (the ventral posterior nucleus), synapsing upon third-order neurones that project to the somatosensory cortex in the postcentral gyrus of the parietal lobe. Throughout the central projections of the somatosensory system there is a high degree of spatial segregation of the neurones representing different parts of the body (so-called somatotopic

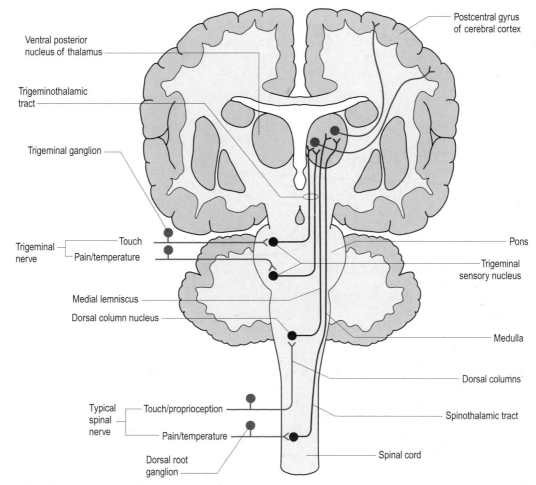

Fig. 1.26 **Overview of major pathways for general sensation.** First-order neurones are green, second-order neurones are red and third-order neurones are blue.

organisation). This is most dramatically demonstrated at the level of the cerebral cortex. Here the somatosensory area occupies a strip of cortex that extends from the medial aspect of the hemisphere (leg area) to the inferolateral aspect of the parietal lobe (head area).

The major motor pathways

The motor neurones that directly innervate skeletal muscle have cell bodies lying in the grey matter of the spinal cord and brain stem and are often referred to as **lower motor neurones**. They constitute the final common pathway by which the nervous system controls movement. In contrast, the neurones forming the descending tracts, which control the activity of lower motor neurones, are themselves collectively referred to as **upper motor neurones**. There are a number of such descending tracts, the **corticospinal** and **corticobulbar tracts** being among the most important (Fig. 1.27). These originate partly from neurones in the motor area of the cerebral cortex, where the whole body is represented in a somatotopic fashion. Axons pass through the internal capsule and into the brain stem, where most of them decussate to the other side. This means that movements of one side of the body are controlled by the opposite cerebral cortex. Corticobulbar fibres control the activity of motor neurones located in cranial nerve nuclei, which innervate skeletal muscles of the head and neck through the cranial nerves. Corticospinal fibres control the activity of motor neurones in the spinal cord, which innervate trunk and limb muscles. The place where corticospinal fibres cross over to the other side of the

nervous system can be seen on the ventral aspect of the medulla (Fig. 9.5) and is known as the **decussation of the pyramids**. Because of this, the corticospinal tract is also known as the **pyramidal tract**.

The main function of the corticobulbar and corticospinal pathways is the control of voluntary, skilled movements. A large proportion of the motor cortex and its descending pathways are, therefore, devoted to those parts of the body capable of delicate, fractionated movements, such as the muscles of speech and facial expression and the muscles controlling the hand.

Numerous brain structures apart from the corticospinal or pyramidal system are involved in the control of movement, posture and muscle tone; these are sometimes collectively known as **extrapyramidal** pathways. They include certain nuclei in the brain stem, such as the **vestibular nuclei** and the **reticular nuclei** (reticular formation), and also the **basal ganglia** and related subcortical nuclei located in the forebrain. The vestibular and reticular nuclei influence spinal motor neurones through descending connections in the vestibulospinal and reticulospinal tracts. They are important in the control of muscle tone and the posture of the body. The basal ganglia exert their actions on the lower motor neurones of the brain stem and spinal cord of the contralateral side through complex, indirect pathways (Fig. 1.28). These include projections via the thalamus to the motor areas of the cerebral cortex and projections to the reticular formation of the brain stem. The basal ganglia are important in the facilitation of appropriate motor behaviour and the inhibition of unwanted movements.

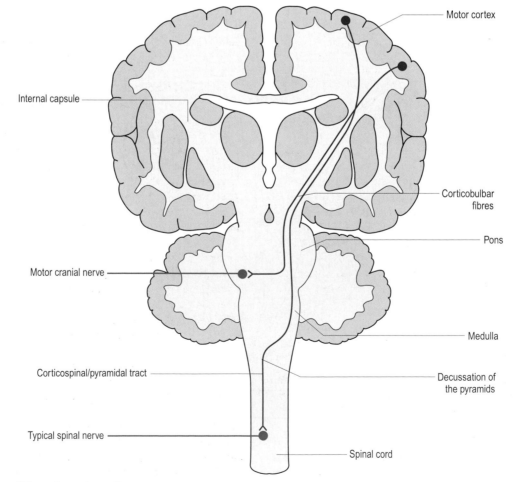

Fig. 1.27 **Overview of the major motor pathways.**

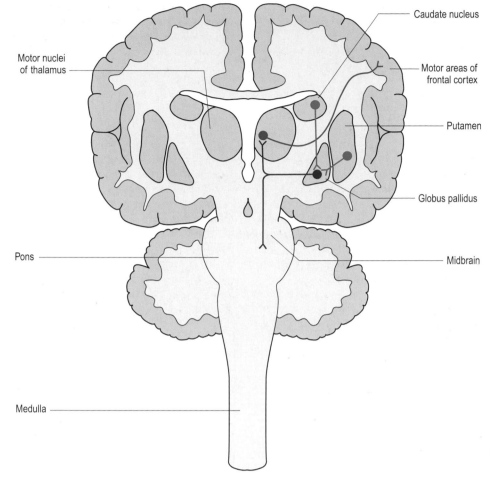

Caudate nucleus

Motor nuclei of thalamus

Motor areas of frontal cortex

Putamen

Globus pallidus

Pons

Midbrain

Medulla

Fig. 1.28 **Overview of the connections of the basal ganglia.**

The cerebellum is an important centre in which programmes of movement, generated in the motor region of the cerebral cortex, are compared with sensory feedback concerning the speed and direction of active movements of the limbs, head and neck in space. This is essential for accurate, coordinated, purposeful movement. The cerebellum receives afferent connections from the spinal cord in the spinocerebellar tracts and from the motor cortex. Its efferent connections are complex but are primarily in the form of feedback to the thalamus and thence to the motor cortex (Fig. 1.29). Afferents to each side of the cerebellum come from the ipsilateral half of the spinal cord and from the contralateral cerebral cortex. Efferent projections are directed to the contralateral thalamus and cerebral cortex through a decussation in the midbrain. Because of the decussation of cortical descending motor pathways, each side of the cerebellum, therefore, coordinates the movements of the ipsilateral side of the body.

Basic clinical diagnostic principles

A knowledge of neuroanatomy is a prerequisite for the clinical diagnosis of disorders of the nervous system. The process of diagnosis proceeds by history-taking, by the neurological examination and finally by confirmatory investigations (Fig. 1.30). History-taking provides clues to the aetiology or cause of disease, whereas the clinical examination pinpoints the site of the lesion (Fig. 1.31). A pathological lesion acting at a specific locality within the neuromuscular axis forms a

recognisable syndrome, investigation of which leads to establishing the aetiology or diagnosis.

Aetiology of neurological disease

The disorders of the neuromuscular system are of four major types (Fig. 1.32) in relation to causation or aetiology.

For each major cause of disease there are appropriate types of investigation leading to specific forms of treatment. The four causes are ranked in order of clinical priority so that conditions that are common, potentially life-threatening and reversible with prompt treatment are either established or excluded first. Conditions that are rare, chronic and incurable can be considered later.

Extrinsic disorders

Extrinsic disorders lead to compression of the brain, spinal cord, nerve roots and peripheral nerves (Fig. 1.33) and are, therefore, surgically remediable. Investigations, such as the neuroradiological imaging of the central nervous system, must be promptly carried out prior to neurosurgical intervention. Delay in decompressive neurosurgery can lead to permanent paralysis, sensory loss and incontinence.

The cerebrum, spinal cord and peripheral nerves can be compressed by disease of adjacent structures. The brain may be compressed on its outer surface by blood clots (**haematomas**), abscesses and tumours arising within the skull and coverings of the cerebrum. Alternatively, the fluid-filled ventricles may compress the brain from within when blockage to the flow of CSF leads to a rise in pressure and expansion of the ventricles (**hydrocephalus**).

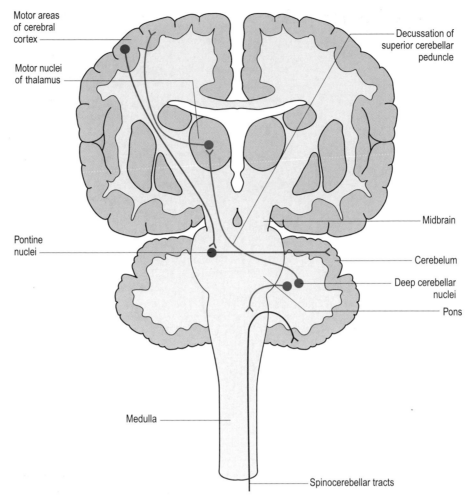

Fig. 1.29 **Overview of the connections of the cerebellum.**

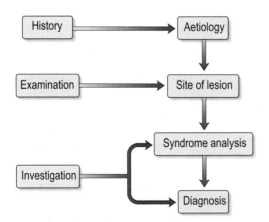

Fig. 1.30 **The process of clinical diagnosis.**

The spinal cord may be compressed by disease of the spine, such as arthritis (**spondylosis**), prolapsed intervertebral discs and bone tumours, as well as by tumours of the meninges (**meningiomas**). The central canal of the spinal cord, normally a minute vestigial space, may expand into a cavity (**syrinx**), compressing the nerve fibres in the centre of the cord (**syringomyelia**).

The cranial nerves emerging from the brain stem may be compressed as they course through the cranium and leave the foramina of the skull by tumours and swollen arteries (**aneurysms**). The spinal nerve roots leaving the spinal cord

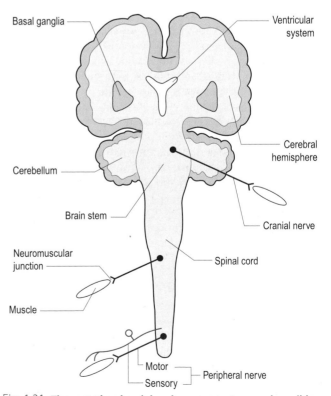

Fig. 1.31 **The central and peripheral nervous systems and possible sites of pathological lesion.**

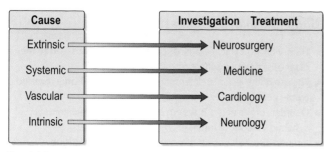

Fig. 1.32 **The four major categories of disorders of the neuromuscular system.**

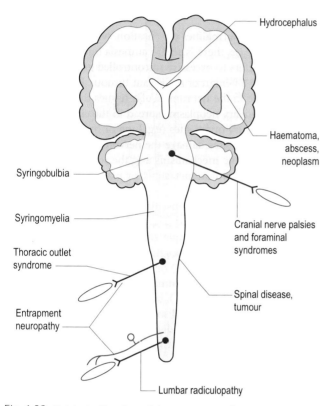

Fig. 1.33 **Extrinsic disorders of the neuromuscular system.**

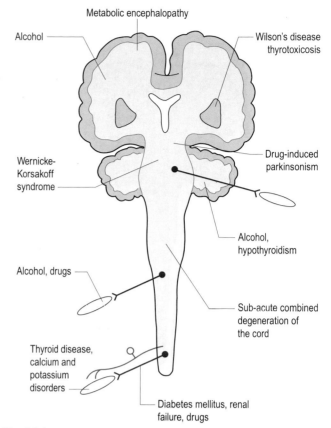

Fig. 1.34 **Systemic disorders of the neuromuscular system.**

in the neck and back may be trapped by tumours and prolapsed intervertebral discs, causing pain, weakness and sensory loss in their region of distribution (**radiculopathy**). The peripheral nerves may become trapped at vulnerable pressure sites in the limbs by ribs and tough fibrous bands, leading to pain, weakness and sensory loss in their distribution (**entrapment neuropathy**).

Investigations for extrinsic disorders are chiefly neuroradiological (e.g. computed tomographic (CT) brain scan, magnetic resonance imaging (MRI)) to delineate the disorders (lesions) for neurosurgical decompression. Surgery may be required urgently to prevent permanent disability and that is why extrinsic disorders should be the first diagnostic consideration.

Systemic disorders

Systemic disorders are primarily of organs other than the nervous system but disrupt neuromuscular function by abnormal metabolism (Fig. 1.34). The patient presents with a neurological condition or syndrome, but the cause lies primarily elsewhere. It may be intoxication with drugs (for example, alcohol), dietary deficiency (for example, vitamin B), failure of the cardiorespiratory system, liver or kidneys,

or hormonal (endocrine) disorders such as thyroid disease, diabetes mellitus and abnormalities in calcium and potassium balance. Investigations for systemic disease are chiefly haematological, biochemical tests and specific measures of cardiorespiratory, liver, renal and endocrine function. Treatment of the systemic disease by the appropriate specialist can lead to cure of the neurological disorder.

Vascular disorders

Vascular disorders (Fig. 1.35) damage the circulation to the nervous system in a number of ways:

- occlusion of the vessels (**thrombosis**)
- restricting the blood and oxygen supply (**infarction**)
- bleeding into the nervous tissues (**haemorrhage**).

The rapid development of a vascular lesion is called a **stroke**. Congenital swellings of arteries (**aneurysms**) or tumours of blood vessels (**angiomas**) can compress cranial nerves and the brain itself. Investigations for vascular disorders are aimed at excluding abnormal clotting disorders of the circulating blood, testing the valves and muscles of the heart (echocardiography, electrocardiography and cardiac angiography), and displaying the vessels of the neck and brain by angiography. The treatment of vascular disorders may be haematological or cardiological and may require surgery to the heart or arteries in the neck and skull.

Intrinsic disorders

Intrinsic disorders (Fig. 1.36) are primary disorders of the nervous system itself. Intrinsic primary neurological disorders are uncommon and often chronic and irreversible, so that a more leisurely series of investigations can be chosen. Many nervous disorders are under genetic influences

Major motor pathways

The fact that the descending motor pathways in the corticobulbar and corticospinal tracts decussate in the lower brain stem accounts for the observation that a unilateral lesion in the cerebral hemisphere (Fig. 13.19) or brain stem (Fig. 9.14) leads to contralateral paralysis of the limbs. This stands in contrast to a unilateral lesion in the spinal cord which causes ipsilateral limb paralysis (Fig. 8.21E). It is important to recognise that the descending motor pathways, or upper motor neurones, despite being highly organised somatotopically, are concerned primarily with concerted movements of the limbs. Damage to these pathways (upper motor neurone lesion) leads to a breakdown in movements of extension and abduction of the upper limbs and of flexion of the lower limbs. This characteristic weakness of movements is clinically referred to as a **pyramidal weakness**.

Pyramidal weakness is characterised by increased tone, i.e. resistance to passive limb movement, termed **spasticity**. The increase in tone occurs at the initial stretch of the limb muscles and is then followed by relaxation of tone (clasp-knife response). Spasticity manifests in the flexor muscles of the upper limbs and extensor muscles of the lower limbs. These are also the stronger muscle groups in the respective limbs, and the combination of spasticity and greater power contributes to the development of an abnormal posture in which the arms are relatively fixed in flexion and the legs in extension (Fig. 13.19).

The motor neurones arising in the brain stem and forming the cranial nerves, together with those leaving the ventral horns of the spinal cord in the motor roots of spinal nerves, are lower motor neurones and innervate specific muscle fibres. Damage to lower motor neurones therefore leads to weakness and wasting of individual muscles, as opposed to disruption of whole integrated movements. The muscles lose their tone (**hypotonia**). Autonomous, spontaneous contractions of the muscle fibres associated with a single motor nerve (motor unit) occur when the muscle fibres are denervated and are seen as **fasciculations**, i.e. ripple-like movements of muscle beneath the skin.

Lower and upper motor neurone syndromes

Damage to lower motor neurones is associated with a number of motor signs and symptoms that distinguish it from upper motor neurone lesions. The distinction between lower and upper motor neurone syndromes is critical in neurological examination and diagnosis. The clinical signs of damage to the upper neurone functions are often referred to as **pyramidal signs**.

Lower motor neurone syndrome

- Weakness (paresis) or paralysis (plegia) of individual muscles.
- Wasting of muscles
- Visible spontaneous contractions of motor units (fasciculation)
- Reduced resistance to passive stretching (hypotonia)
- Diminution or loss of deep tendon reflexes (hyporeflexia or areflexia).

Upper motor neurone syndrome

- Weakness or paralysis of specific movements (extension of the upper limbs and flexion of the lower limbs, termed 'pyramidal weakness')
- No wasting of muscles
- Increased resistance to passive stretching of muscles (spasticity); initial resistance to muscular stretching followed by relaxation (clasp-knife response)
- Hyperactivity of deep tendon reflexes (hyperreflexia)
- Emergence of the extensor plantar response (positive **Babinski reflex**) leading to dorsiflexion of the great toe on stimulation of the sole of the foot.

Because of the decussation of the principal motor pathways in the lower brain stem, lesions located in the cerebral hemispheres and higher brain stem cause paralysis of the limbs opposite (contralateral) to the side of the lesion, whereas spinal cord lesions lead to paralysis of the limbs on the same side as (ipsilateral to) the lesion.

The term 'pyramidal signs' implies that these clinical features result solely from damage to the pyramidal, or corticospinal, tract. However, individual tracts are rarely damaged in isolation and, therefore, it is often difficult to attribute clinical deficits to involvement of particular pathways. Damage to the pyramidal tract itself probably accounts for the loss of discrete movements and the appearance of the Babinski reflex. Hyperreflexia and spasticity are due to the involvement of other pathways.

Cerebellar pathways

The plan of an intended movement is transmitted to the cerebellum from the motor parts of the cerebral cortex and the basal ganglia via the brain stem. Once the specific movement takes place, afferent stimuli from sensory receptors of the limbs, conveying information about the actual movement, flow through the peripheral nerves into the spinal cord and ascend in the spinocerebellar tracts, via the brain stem to the cerebellum. The cerebellum, therefore, is in a unique position to compare the intended with the actual movements of the limbs in space. When there is a discrepancy between these, the cerebellum is able to correct deviant movements. This is achieved by ascending pathways travelling via the thalamus to the motor cortex and thence through descending fibres passing to the brain stem and spinal cord. There are also direct cerebellar connections to the vestibular and reticular nuclei of the brain stem.

Lesions of the cerebellar pathways lead to **incoordination of movements**, or **ataxia**, of the head, neck and limbs in the absence of weakness or loss of sensation. The lesion interrupting the cerebellar pathways may lie in the cerebellum itself, the brain stem or the ascending spinocerebellar pathways in the spinal cord. Unilateral lesions of the cerebellum lead to ipsilateral loss of coordination. Similarly, a unilateral lesion of the brain stem inevitably destroys the cerebellar connections to the cerebral hemisphere and spinal cord and leads to ipsilateral incoordination and, as described above, a contralateral pyramidal weakness of the limbs.

It is sometimes mistakenly thought that incoordination of the limbs is synonymous with a disorder of the cerebellum. This is not the case, whereas it is true that lesions of the cerebellum do lead to incoordination. A patient with a short leg and an arthritic hip joint, for example, will have an incoordinate gait. Moreover, weakness of the limbs due to

> ## Disorders of the cerebellum
> Disease of the cerebellum leads to a **cerebellar syndrome** comprising incoordination of eye movements (nystagmus), speech (dysarthria), the upper limbs (intention tremor) and gait (ataxia). The symptoms and signs occur on the same side as (ipsilateral to) the lesion in the cerebellum.

disease of the central or peripheral nervous system will cause incoordination. Damage to the peripheral sensory nerves or to the dorsal columns of the spinal cord deprives the brain of proprioceptive information from the limbs, thus causing lack of coordination of the arms and an ataxic gait. This is known as 'sensory ataxia'. When patients with sensory ataxia close their eyes they readily lose their balance and this is known as Romberg's sign. This does not happen with lesions of the cerebellar pathways.

Because of these problems of interpretation it is conventional to carry out tasks of coordination at the end of the neurological examination in order to assess the contribution of orthopaedic deformities, neurological weakness and sensory loss to the degree of incoordination. If these prior deficits can be excluded on examination then incoordination can reliably be blamed on lesions of the cerebellar pathways themselves. This can sometimes be a difficult exercise; for example, in diseases such as multiple sclerosis, there are multiple lesions in the cerebellum, brain stem and spinal cord, each making a contribution to the nature and degree of neurological disability.

Basal ganglia

The basal ganglia, lying deep within the cerebral hemisphere, receive sensory and motor information from all parts of the cerebral cortex and also from the brain stem and spinal cord. Their functions are difficult to describe succinctly but they may be regarded as structures which facilitate useful, purposeful movements and inhibit unwanted movements. They are also important in the control of posture and muscle tone. These functions are illustrated by the symptoms of basal ganglia dysfunction, which cover a wide spectrum of manifestations. Lesions of the basal ganglia do not lead to loss of sensation, power or coordination. Instead, there is a loss of control over voluntary movements and posture, alterations in muscle tone and the emergence of abnormal involuntary movements (**dyskinesia**). Unilateral lesions of the basal ganglia lead to a contralateral motor disorder.

In Parkinson's disease, for example, there is slowness in the initiation and execution of movement (**akinesia, bradykinesia, hypokinesia**). There is a characteristic slow, rhythmic **tremor** at rest. There is also increased tone (**hypertonia, rigidity**) of the limbs. Rigidity is characteristic of basal ganglia disorders and is manifest as resistance to passive movement throughout the whole excursion of the limb. It differs from spasticity, in which there is an initial resistance to passive movement of the limb, followed by relaxation (see above). In some forms of basal ganglia disease muscular tone is reduced (**hypotonia**).

In contrast, in Huntington's disease and levodopa-induced dyskinesia, there appear abnormal involuntary movements which take the form of inappropriate, quasi-purposeful

> ## Disorders of the basal ganglia
> Disorders of the basal ganglia do not cause paralysis or sensory loss but lead to abnormal control of movement and posture and changes in muscular tone. There may be slowness in the initiation and execution of movement (hypokinesia, bradykinesia, akinesia), or abnormal 'involuntary' movements (dyskinesia, hyperkinesia) may appear. Where increased muscle tone is present, the increased resistance to passive stretching of muscles occurs throughout the act of stretching and is described by clinicians as **rigidity**. Rigidity is distinguished from **spasticity**; the latter is associated with pyramidal weakness and hyperreflexia, which are not found in the extrapyramidal syndrome. Disorders of the basal ganglia cause symptoms on the opposite (contralateral) side of the body.

fragments of normal movement (**chorea**). The slow serpentine twisting of the limbs in idiopathic **dystonia** contrasts with the sudden shock-like muscle jerks of **myoclonus** and the brief stereotypical repetitive movements of **tics**.

Neuropsychological functions

The neuropsychological functions of language, perception, spatial analysis, learned skilled movements, memory and problem-solving (or executive functions) are organised within the cerebral hemispheres (Fig. 1.44). Accordingly, lesions of the brain stem, cerebellum and spinal cord are not accompanied by psychological deficits.

The organisation of neuropsychological functions within the cerebral hemisphere is highly localised, as with the motor and sensory systems (Fig. 13.1).

Language functions (speech, reading, writing and calculation) are organised in the regions of the frontal, parietal and temporal lobes adjacent to the left lateral fissure, the so-called 'language area'. Whereas primary visual processes are organised in the occipital lobes, the **perception** or recognition of objects and human faces is organised in projections to the temporal lobes of the brain. The spatial ability to navigate the limbs and body in space (**visuospatial function**) is organised through projections to

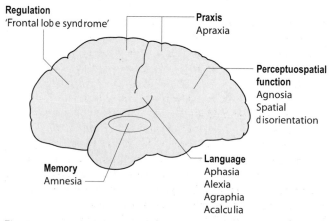

Fig. 1.44 **Regional localisation of neuropsychological functions in the cerebral hemisphere and the syndromes associated with dysfunction.**

the parietal lobes. The premotor areas of the frontal lobes, including the supplementary motor area which lies on the medial aspect of the hemisphere, govern the enactment of learned, skilled movements of the head, neck and limbs (**praxis**). Structures in the medial aspects of the temporal lobes, part of the limbic system, are responsible for learning new information and recollecting from experience (**memory**). The organisation of behaviour involving problem-solving and the achievement of goal-directed behaviour (**executive function**) is organised within the prefrontal areas of the frontal lobes.

It can be deduced from these neuropsychological and anatomical correlations that lesions of the language area will lead to loss of speech (**aphasia**), reading (**alexia**), writing (**agraphia**) and calculation (**acalculia**), whereas lesions of the temporo-parietal cortex lead to loss of perception (**agnosia**) and spatial orientation (**visuospatial disorientation**). Loss of the knowledge of learned skilled movements (**apraxia**) follows lesions of the premotor cortex. Bilateral disorders of the medial temporal lobes and limbic system lead to loss of memory function (**amnesia**). Damage to the prefrontal cortex leads to marked behavioural disturbance with loss of forethought, planning and appropriate affect, manifest in a marked change of personality and behaviour (**frontal lobe** or **dysexecutive syndrome**).

Investigation of neuromuscular disease

The clinical definition of a particular syndrome permits the choice of appropriate investigations to confirm the diagnosis. The major focus of investigations involves:

- CSF analysis
- neuroradiology
- neurophysiology
- neuropathology (biopsy).

Lumbar puncture enables the measurement of CSF pressure and the collection of CSF for bacteriological, biochemical, serological and cytological analyses. These may reveal the presence of blood (**subarachnoid haemorrhage**), infection, immune disease such as multiple sclerosis or the presence of tumour cells.

Neuroradiology encompasses conventional X-ray imaging of the skull and vertebral column, structural imaging of the brain and spinal cord (**computed tomography** and **magnetic resonance imaging**)

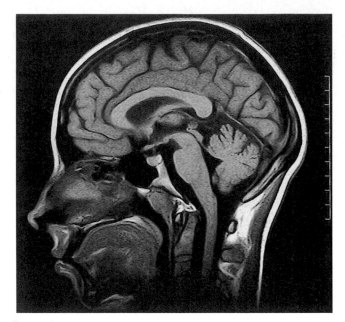

Fig. 1.45 **T$_1$-weighted magnetic resonance image of the brain.**
(Courtesy of Professor A Jackson)

(Fig. 1.45) and functional imaging of cerebral blood flow and metabolism (**single photon emission tomography** (SPECT) and **positron emission tomography** (PET)).

In contrast radiology, an opaque medium is injected into the arteries or veins (**angiography**) to delineate the blood vessels, or into the spinal canal (**myelography**) to outline the spinal cord and nerve roots.

Neurophysiology addresses the electrical activity of the CNS by **electroencephalography** (EEG) and the detection and measurement of **evoked responses** to visual, auditory and somatosensory stimuli. **Central magnetic stimulation** to the brain enables measurement of the motor conduction time to the spinal cord and limb muscles. In the peripheral nervous system, measures of motor and sensory **nerve conduction velocity** and evoked **sensory action potentials** are combined with measurement of individual muscle responses to voluntary and electrically evoked contraction (**electromyography**).

The **biopsy** of nerve, muscle and brain tissue sheds light on the pathophysiological process (e.g. axonal degeneration, demyelination, muscular degeneration) and on the aetiology (e.g. inflammation, neoplasia).

Chapter 2
Cells of the nervous system

The principal functional unit of the nervous system is the nerve cell or neurone. These cells are highly specialised for the encoding, conduction and transmission of information. Present in even larger numbers are neuroglial cells, or glia. These do not take part directly in information processing but are, none the less, crucial for normal neural function. Other cells are also present in the nervous system, such as those forming the walls of blood vessels but, unlike neurones and neuroglia, these are not unique to the nervous system.

The neurone

Size and structure
The main structural features, common to all neurones, have been described briefly in Chapter 1. There are, however,

numerous variations of the basic plan. The size of the cell body varies considerably depending upon location and function. For example, some interneurones in the CNS have cell bodies as small as 5 μm in diameter, while the cell bodies of motor neurones innervating striated muscle may exceed 100 μm. The size of the cell body is usually correlated with the length of the axon. Therefore, a small interneurone will have a short axon, perhaps only a fraction of a millimetre in length. A large motor neurone will possess a long axon (for example, those passing from the spinal cord to the muscles of the foot have axons about 1 metre in length).

The **dendritic arborisation** of neurones also shows great variation in the number, size and density of branches, which reflects the organisation of afferent inputs to the cell. This is illustrated by considering the dendritic arborisations of, for example, a pyramidal cell in the cerebral cortex and a Purkinje cell in the cerebellar cortex (Fig. 2.1).

Like most other cells, neurones possess a nucleus. This is usually located in the centre of the cell body and contains the chromosomal DNA. The rest of the intracellular space is occupied by cytoplasm, which contains numerous organelles and inclusions (Fig. 2.2). Many of these are common to cells other than neurones but some have particular prominence or significance in neurones. Numerous microscopic clumps of **Nissl granules**, or substance, can usually be seen in

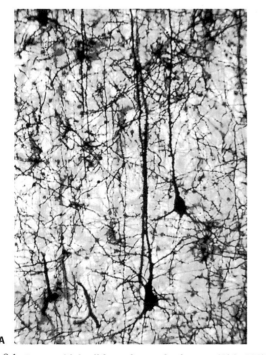
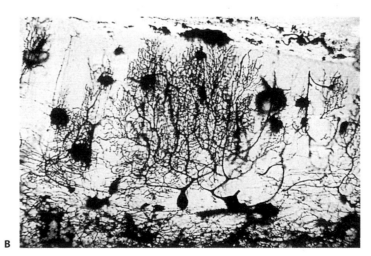

A   B

Fig. 2.1 **A pyramidal cell from the cerebral cortex (A) (× 100) and a Purkinje cell from the cerebellar cortex (B) (× 90) showing the diversity of dendritic arborisations.** Golgi–Cox stain.

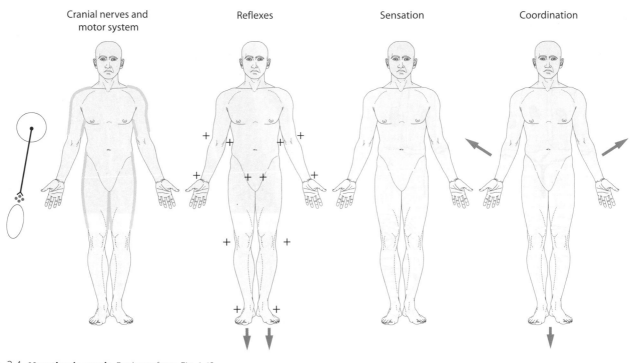

Cranial nerves and motor system | Reflexes | Sensation | Coordination

Fig. 3.4 **Myasthenia gravis.** For key refer to Fig. 1.43.

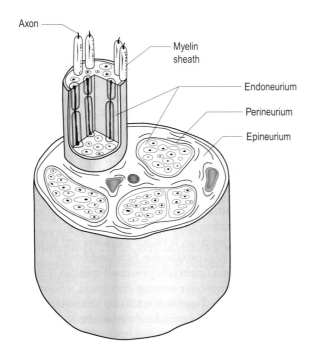

Fig. 3.5 **The structure of a peripheral nerve.**

while the arachnoid and pia are continuous with the perineurium and endoneurium.

Degeneration and regeneration

When a peripheral nerve fibre is transected or otherwise seriously damaged, the portion distal to the transection dies and undergoes degeneration. This is known as **anterograde** or **Wallerian degeneration**. The proximal portion of the neurone, which remains attached to the cell body, may, however, survive and eventually undergo recovery or **regeneration**. The further from the cell body that transection occurs, the more likely it is that the cell body will

survive. Initially, it too usually shows degenerative changes, known as **retrograde degeneration**. This is characterised by dispersal and loss of staining of Nissl substance (chromatolysis), swelling of the cell body and movement of the normally central nucleus to a peripheral location. If the cell recovers, the distal end of the surviving nerve fibre undergoes sprouting. If the two ends of the peripheral nerve are physically aligned, the new regenerating fibres may enter the endoneurial tubes that have lost their nerve fibres. Continued growth of the new fibres, at a rate of 1–2 mm a day, may eventually lead to reinnervation of the original structure and recovery of function. Many factors influence the degree to which successful reinnervation and functional recovery take place.

The degenerative processes that follow nerve cell injury are essentially similar in the CNS. Sprouting of surviving

Peripheral sensorimotor neuropathies

Peripheral sensorimotor neuropathies are characterised by muscular weakness and wasting (especially of distal muscles), distal areflexia and a 'glove and stocking' distribution of sensory loss (Fig. 3.6). Peripheral neuropathies may be caused by systemic disease, vascular disease, heredo-degenerative disorders, infection, immune disorders and paraneoplastic syndromes.

In general, there are two pathological types. **Demyelinating neuropathies** predominantly damage Schwann cells and myelin sheaths. **Axonal neuropathies** primarily cause axonal degeneration. Recovery from neuropathy requires remyelination and regeneration of axons.

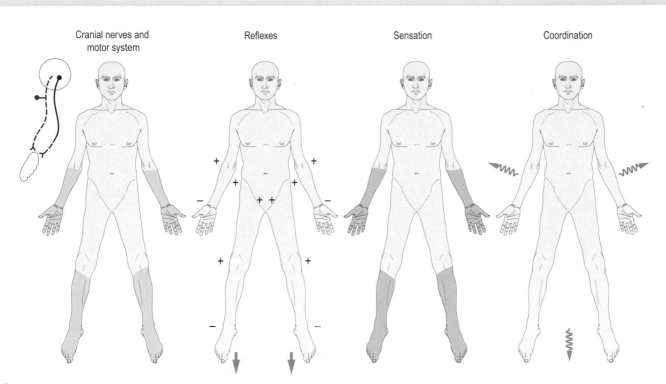

Cranial nerves and motor system | Reflexes | Sensation | Coordination

Fig. 3.6 **Peripheral sensorimotor neuropathy.** For key refer to Fig. 1.43.

neurones also occurs in the CNS, but the re-establishment of previous connections does not, unfortunately, take place to any significant extent.

Distribution of spinal and peripheral nerves

At the roots of the upper and lower limbs are located the brachial plexus (Figs 3.7 and 3.8) and the lumbosacral plexus (Fig. 3.9), respectively. Here, the nerve fibres present in spinal nerves become redistributed to form named peripheral nerves, which then run distally to their targets. The distribution of peripheral nerves is, therefore, different from that of spinal nerves.

Each spinal nerve carries the sensory innervation for a part of the body surface. The area of skin that is supplied by a particular spinal nerve is known as a **dermatome**. Dermatome maps are given in Figure 3.10. These are only approximate, since in reality the cutaneous territories of adjacent spinal nerves overlap considerably. The cutaneous distribution of important peripheral nerves is also illustrated in Figure 3.10.

The group of skeletal muscles innervated by a particular spinal nerve is collectively known as a **myotome**. These muscles are usually functionally related and are responsible for particular patterns of movement. The segmental spinal nerve values of some important movements are shown in Figure 3.11.

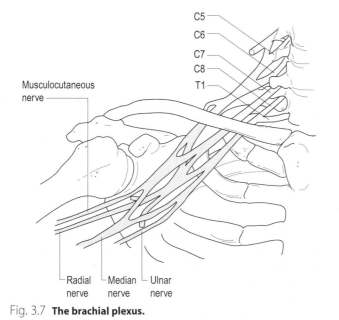

Musculocutaneous nerve

C5
C6
C7
C8
T1

Radial nerve   Median nerve   Ulnar nerve

Fig. 3.7 **The brachial plexus.**

Brachial plexus lesions

In motorcycle accidents, trauma to the shoulder and neck may cause **avulsion of the brachial plexus**, causing immediate weakness and loss of feeling in one upper limb. Later, the arm wastes and becomes painful.

A tumour of the apex of the lung may infiltrate the lower part of the brachial plexus, producing severe pain in the arm, weakness and wasting of the hand and sensory loss on the inner aspect of the forearm and hand (**Pancoast's syndrome**).

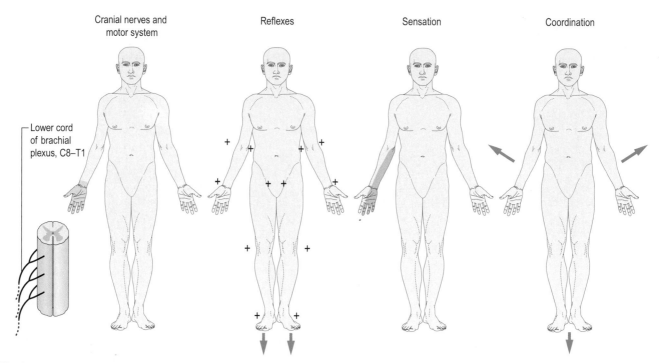

Cranial nerves and motor system · Reflexes · Sensation · Coordination

Lower cord of brachial plexus, C8–T1

Fig. 3.8 **Brachial plexus lesion.** For key refer to Fig. 1.43.

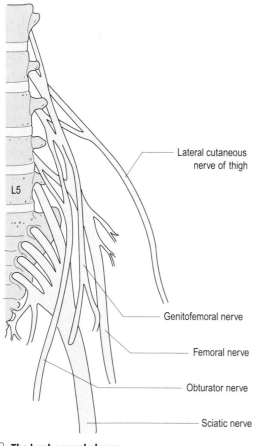

L5

Lateral cutaneous nerve of thigh

Genitofemoral nerve

Femoral nerve

Obturator nerve

Sciatic nerve

Fig. 3.9 **The lumbosacral plexus.**

Lumbosacral plexus lesions
Malignant disease and surgical procedures for cancer can damage the lumbosacral plexus in its course through the pelvis, causing pain, weakness and wasting of the muscles and numbness of the leg(s), with bladder and bowel incontinence.

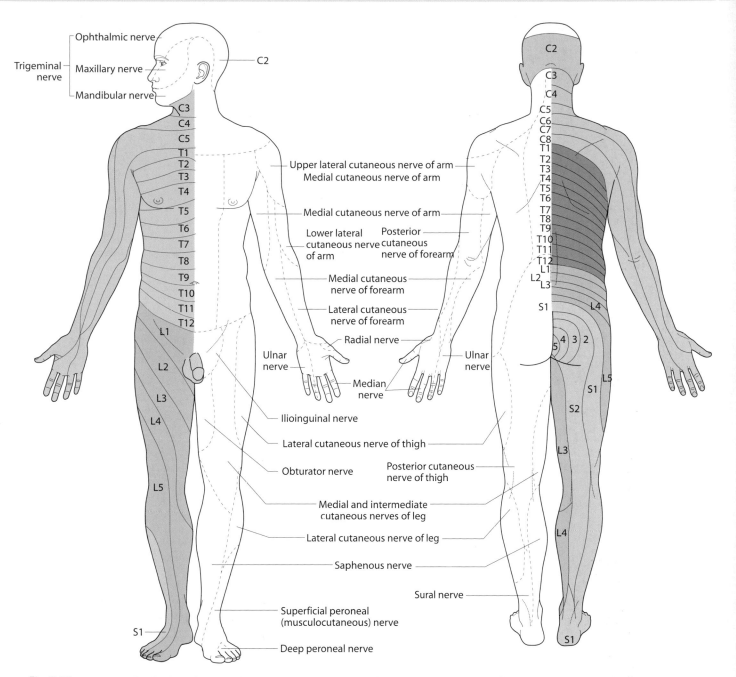

Fig. 3.10 **Cutaneous distribution of (right) spinal nerves (dermatomes) and named peripheral nerves (left).** The cutaneous distribution of the three divisions of the trigeminal nerve is also illustrated.

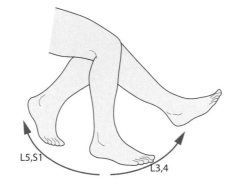
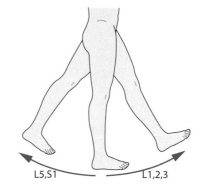
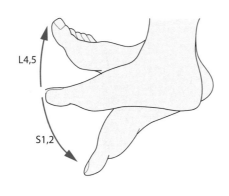
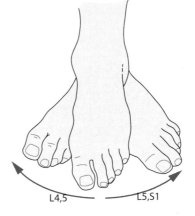

A

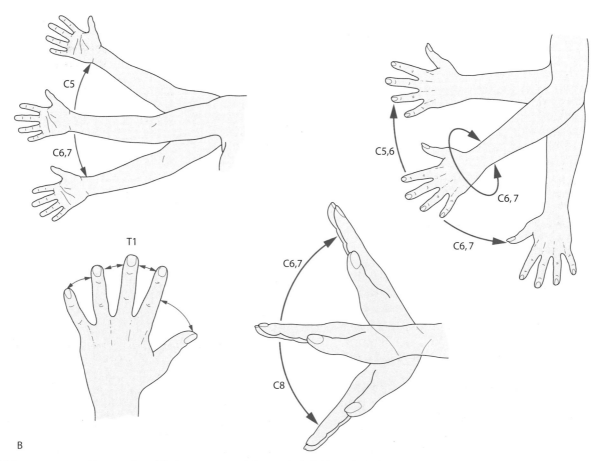

B

Fig. 3.11 **The segmental innervation of limb movements. (A)** Upper limb; **(B)** lower limb.

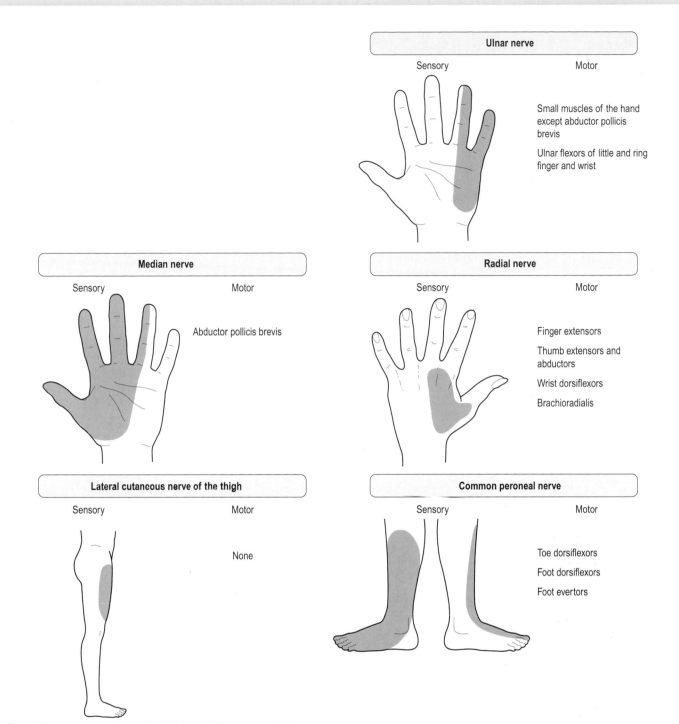

Fig. 3.12 **Sensory and motor deficits in peripheral nerve lesions.**

Compression and entrapment neuropathies

Peripheral nerves are vulnerable to extrinsic compression (e.g. excessive pressure on a recumbent limb) and to chronic entrapment by normal or diseased anatomical structures adjacent to them. The most common examples are **radial nerve** compression in the spiral groove of the humerus, and chronic entrapment of the **ulnar nerve** at the elbow and of the **median nerve** at the wrist (carpal tunnel syndrome) in the upper limb. Entrapment of the **lateral cutaneous nerve of the thigh** and compression of the **common peroneal nerve** at the head of the fibula occur in the lower limb (Fig. 3.12).

Peripheral nerves

- Peripheral nerves consist of variable numbers of bundles, or fascicles, of nerve fibres.
- Fibres are ensheathed in three connective tissue coverings: endoneurium, perineurium and epineurium.
- The endoneurial tubes within which individual axons lie are important for successful regeneration and reinnervation by nerves following nerve injury.
- Many nerve fibres in cranial and spinal nerves become rearranged as they course peripherally, by passage through nerve plexuses.
- The area of skin supplied by a spinal nerve is called a dermatome.
- The group of muscles innervated by a spinal nerve is called a myotome.

Chapter 4
Autonomic nervous system

The term autonomic nervous system is used to describe those nerve cells, located within both the central and peripheral nervous systems, that are concerned with the innervation and control of visceral organs, smooth muscle and secretory glands. The principal function of the autonomic nervous system is broadly described as homeostasis of the internal environment. This is achieved by regulation of cardiovascular, respiratory, digestive, excretory and thermoregulatory mechanisms, which occurs automatically and with relatively little volitional control.

Autonomic afferent and efferent fibres enter and leave the CNS through spinal and cranial nerves. Within the spinal cord and brain stem they establish interconnections through which autonomic reflexes are mediated. Afferent fibres also establish connections with ascending neurones through which conscious awareness of visceral function is achieved. Changes in the internal and external environment, and emotional factors, profoundly influence autonomic activity, most notably via descending connections from the **hypothalamus**. Autonomic efferent neurones differ from those of the somatic nervous system in that there is a sequence of two neurones between the CNS and the innervated structure (Fig. 4.1). The cell body of the first neurone is located in the spinal cord or brain stem, while that of the second neurone is located peripherally in an

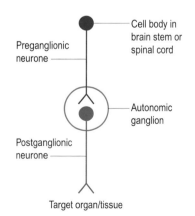

Fig. 4.1 **Basic organisation of the autonomic nervous system into preganglionic and postganglionic neurones.** In the sympathetic division, ganglia constitute the sympathetic chain. Preganglionic neurones, therefore, have relatively short axons, while postganglionic fibres are relatively long. In the parasympathetic division, ganglia are located close to the target organ. Consequently, preganglionic axons are long and postganglionic axons are short.

Table 4.1 **Autonomic nervous system**

Structure	Sympathetic effect	Parasympathetic effect
Iris of eye	Dilates pupil	Constricts pupil
Ciliary muscle of eye	Relaxes	Contracts
Salivary glands	Reduces secretion	Increases secretion
Lacrimal gland	Reduces secretion	Increases secretion
Heart	Increases rate and force of contraction	Decreases rate and force of contraction
Bronchi	Dilates	Constricts
Gastrointestinal tract	Decreases motility	Increases motility
Sweat glands	Increases secretion	
Erector pili muscles	Contracts	

autonomic ganglion. The first neurone is referred to as the **preganglionic neurone** and the second as the **postganglionic neurone**.

The efferent neurones of the autonomic nervous system fall into two distinct anatomical and functional groups or divisions: namely, **sympathetic** and **parasympathetic**. Many, though not all, structures that receive autonomic fibres are dually innervated by both sympathetic and parasympathetic systems. These exercise antagonistic effects upon the innervated structure (Table 4.1).

Sympathetic division

Preganglionic sympathetic neurones are located exclusively in the thoracic and upper two or three lumbar segments of the spinal cord (Fig. 4.2). They lie in the **lateral horn** of the spinal grey matter, which is, therefore, only present at these levels (see Figs 8.8 and 8.9). Preganglionic axons leave the cord in the ventral nerve root and join the spinal nerve. Postganglionic sympathetic neurones have their cell bodies in one of two locations: either the **sympathetic chain** of ganglia that lies alongside the vertebral column, or the plexuses (coeliac, superior mesenteric, inferior mesenteric) that surround the main branches of the abdominal aorta. In order to reach either of these locations, preganglionic axons in the spinal nerve enter the sympathetic chain. Ganglia of the sympathetic chain are linked to those spinal nerves which contain sympathetic outflow by two small nerves, the **rami communicantes** (Fig. 4.3). Preganglionic fibres pass into the chain via the white ramus communicantes, so called because the fibres are myelinated.

Those fibres concerned with innervation of structures in the head and thorax terminate in synaptic contact with postganglionic cell bodies in the sympathetic chain. The postganglionic fibres return to the spinal nerve via the grey ramus communicantes, so called because the fibres are contribute to the myenteric (Auerbach's) and submucosal (Meissner's) plexuses.

These plexuses are also referred to as the 'enteric nervous system'. Such a concept has arisen because the plexuses additionally contain afferent neurones and interneurones. The rich local interconnections of these cells are capable of sustaining the motility of the gastrointestinal tract in the absence of input from the CNS. Furthermore, these cells cannot simply be equated with the parasympathetic nervous system as traditionally defined, since they are known also to receive synaptic input from postganglionic sympathetic neurones. The neurotransmitter released by both preganglionic and postganglionic parasympathetic neurones is acetylcholine.

Chapter 5
Coverings of the central nervous system

The CNS is supported and protected by bone and membranous coverings. The brain is located within the cranial cavity of the skull and the spinal cord lies in the vertebral, or spinal, canal within the vertebral column, or spine. Within their bony coverings, the brain and spinal cord are invested by three concentric membranous envelopes. The outermost membrane is the **dura mater**, the middle layer is the **arachnoid mater** and the innermost layer is the **pia mater**. The vertebral column and spinal meninges are described in Chapter 8; consequently, only the skull and cranial meninges are considered here.

Skull

The brain lies on the floor of the cranial cavity, which, together with the bones of the cranial vault, provides support and protection from physical injury. The floor of the cranial cavity consists of three **fossae**. Each of these accommodates particular parts of the brain and possesses **foramina**

Raised intracranial pressure
A **space-occupying lesion** is an expanding focal lesion such as a tumour, haematoma or abscess. Since the cranial cavity is closed and unyielding, the brain is distorted and displaced downwards, towards the foramen magnum, as the intracranial pressure rises. The patient complains of headache, vomiting, blurring of vision and drowsiness. The optic discs are swollen (**papilloedema**), signs of brain stem dysfunction are found, and coma and death supervene if the pressure is not relieved by neurosurgery (craniotomy). **Benign intracranial hypertension** is caused by generalised swelling of the brain in the absence of a focal space-occupying lesion. It often occurs in obese young women; the syndrome of raised intracranial pressure mimics a brain tumour, hence the old designation, 'pseudo tumour cerebri'.

through which cranial nerves and blood vessels enter and leave the cranial cavity (Fig. 5.1).

Anterior cranial fossa
The anterior cranial fossa is formed by the frontal, ethmoid and sphenoid bones. It contains the frontal lobes of the brain. The greater part of the floor of the anterior cranial fossa consists of the frontal bone and it also forms the roof of the orbit. The part of the frontal bone that forms the anterior wall of the fossa contains the **frontal air sinus**. In the midline of the floor of the anterior cranial fossa is the ethmoid bone. In the midline a sharp ridge, the crista galli, provides attachment for the falx cerebri. In a depression on either side of the crista galli lie the **cribriform plates** of the ethmoid. These accommodate the **olfactory bulbs**. The bone of the cribriform plate is peppered with small perforations through which the fascicles of the olfactory nerve enter the cranial cavity from the nasal cavity to attach to the olfactory bulb.

Middle cranial fossa
The middle cranial fossa is formed by the sphenoid and temporal bones. In the midline, the body of the sphenoid forms a deep depression, the **hypophyseal fossa**, encompassed by four spurs of bone, the anterior and posterior clinoid processes. In the hypophyseal fossa lies the **hypophysis**, or **pituitary gland**. Lateral to the body of the sphenoid, the rest of the middle cranial fossa contains the temporal lobes of the cerebral hemisphere. The middle cranial fossa contains numerous points of entry and exit from the cranial cavity for cranial nerves and blood vessels.

- The **optic canal** is located medial to the anterior clinoid process and communicates with the orbit. Through it pass the optic (II) nerve and the ophthalmic artery (a branch of the internal carotid artery).
- The **superior orbital fissure** lies between the greater and lesser wings of the sphenoid bone and also communicates with the orbit. It carries the oculomotor (III), trochlear (IV) and abducens (VI) nerves and the ophthalmic division of the trigeminal (V) nerve.
- The **foramen rotundum** opens into the pterygopalatine fossa and carries the maxillary division of the trigeminal nerve.
- The **foramen ovale** carries the large mandibular division of the trigeminal nerve.
- The **foramen lacerum** lies directly beneath the posterior clinoid process. Through this foramen the internal carotid artery enters the cranial cavity.
- The **foramen spinosum** is the point of entry of the middle meningeal artery.

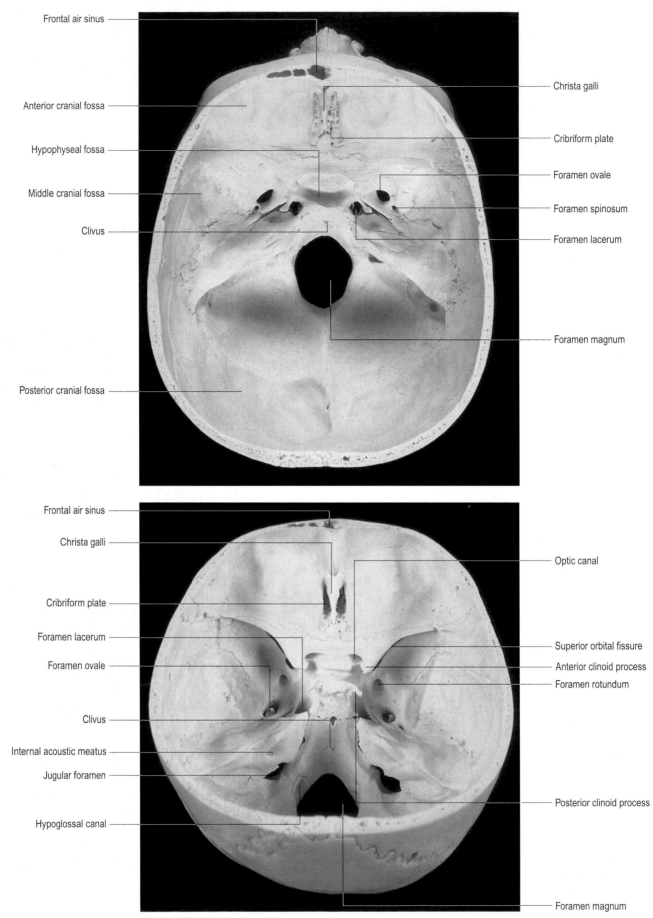

Frontal air sinus

Anterior cranial fossa

Hypophyseal fossa

Middle cranial fossa

Clivus

Posterior cranial fossa

Christa galli

Cribriform plate

Foramen ovale

Foramen spinosum

Foramen lacerum

Foramen magnum

Frontal air sinus

Christa galli

Cribriform plate

Foramen lacerum

Foramen ovale

Clivus

Internal acoustic meatus

Jugular foramen

Hypoglossal canal

Optic canal

Superior orbital fissure

Anterior clinoid process

Foramen rotundum

Posterior clinoid process

Foramen magnum

Fig. 5.1 **Floor of the skull showing the three cranial fossae and principal foramina.**

Foraminal syndromes
The exit foramina of the skull represent sites of potential extrinsic compression of structures running through them, by disorders such as bony deformity and tumours of bone, meninges or blood vessels. The particular cranial nerves damaged at the exit site lead to 'foraminal syndromes', e.g. of the **superior orbital fissure** (see p. 106) or **jugular foramen** (see p. 113). The spinal cord, lower brain stem and the tonsils of the cerebellum are compromised in the **foramen magnum syndrome**.

Posterior cranial fossa

The posterior cranial fossa is formed by the occipital and petrous temporal bones. Anteriorly, in the midline, it forms a steep, smooth slope (the **clivus**) that is continuous with the body of the sphenoid bone, posterior to the hypophyseal fossa. The brain stem rests upon the clivus, the medulla passing through the **foramen magnum** to become continuous with the spinal cord. The foramen magnum also admits the vertebral arteries and the spinal root of the accessory (XI) nerve. In the lateral wall of the foramen magnum lies the **hypoglossal canal** through which the hypoglossal (XII) nerve leaves the cranial cavity. Between the occipital and petrous temporal bones lies the large

---

Skull

- The brain lies on the floor of the cranial cavity, which consists of three fossae.
- The bones of the skull and the meninges provide protection for the brain.
- The anterior cranial fossa contains the frontal lobes of the cerebral hemispheres.
- It forms the roof of the orbit and is closely associated with the frontal air sinus.
- The cribriform plate admits the olfactory nerves to the cranial cavity and accommodates the olfactory bulb.
- The middle cranial fossa contains the temporal lobe. In the midline, the hypophyseal fossa holds the pituitary gland.
- A number of foramina provide entry and exit for important blood vessels and cranial nerves (indicated in parentheses):
  — optic canal (optic nerve, ophthalmic artery)
  — superior orbital fissure (oculomotor, trochlear, abducens and ophthalmic division of trigeminal nerves)
  — foramen rotundum (maxillary division of trigeminal nerve)
  — foramen ovale (mandibular division of trigeminal nerve)
  — foramen lacerum (internal carotid artery)
  — foramen spinosum (middle meningeal artery).
- The posterior cranial fossa accommodates the brain stem and cerebellum.
- A number of important structures pass through the foramina of the posterior fossa:
  — foramen magnum (medulla oblongata, vertebral arteries, spinal root of the accessory nerve)
  — hypoglossal canal (hypoglossal nerve)
  — jugular foramen (internal jugular vein, glossopharyngeal, vagus and accessory nerves)
  — internal auditory meatus (facial and vestibulocochlear nerves).

---

jugular foramen through which pass the internal jugular vein, and the glossopharyngeal (IX), vagus (X) and accessory (XI) nerves. In the vertical wall of the petrous temporal bone is located the **internal auditory (acoustic) meatus**, which transmits the vestibulocochlear (VIII) and facial (VII) nerves. The cerebellum rests on the floor of the posterior cranial fossa.

Cranial meninges

Dura mater

The cranial dura is a tough, fibrous membrane that ensheathes the brain like a loose-fitting bag. In some regions, such as the floor of the cranial cavity and the midline of the cranial roof, the dura is tightly adherent to the interior surface of the skull, while elsewhere, such as the fronto-parietal area, the two are separated by a narrow extradural space. Two large reflections of dura extend into the cranial cavity and occupy the fissures between major components of the brain (Figs 5.2 and 5.3). In the midline, a vertical sheet of dura, the **falx cerebri**, extends from the cranial roof into the great longitudinal fissure between the cerebral hemispheres. The falx, therefore, has an attached border that adheres to the inner surface of the skull and a free border that lies above the corpus callosum. A horizontal shelf of dura, the **tentorium cerebelli**, extends inwards from the occipito-temporal region of the skull to lie in the transverse cerebral fissure, between the posterior part of the cerebral hemispheres and the cerebellum. The tentorium has a free border that encircles the midbrain, as the brain stem communicates between the posterior and middle cranial fossae. In the midline the tentorium becomes continuous superiorly with the falx cerebri.

Head trauma
Head trauma, especially resulting from road traffic accidents, is the most common cause of death and disability in youth. The injury may be blunt ('closed') or caused by a penetrating missile. The skull may be fractured and depressed, tearing brain coverings and the brain itself. Displacement and torsion of the brain lead to contusion, tearing of white matter and bleeding into the brain (**intracerebral haematoma**), causing unconsciousness (concussion), neurological and psychological deficits, and post-traumatic epilepsy.

Tearing of the middle meningeal artery causes bleeding into the extradural space (**extradural haematoma**). As the blood clot expands, the brain is compressed; as a result, coma supervenes a delayed period of hours after the blow. Without neurosurgical evacuation, the rising intracranial pressure causes brain displacement and death.

Tearing of the veins stretching across the subdural space causes gradual seepage of blood, collecting to form a chronic **subdural haematoma** with eventual coma. The delay between the blow and the development of symptoms may be of weeks or months. The elderly are particularly vulnerable and the head injury may be slight and forgotten. Again, surgical removal of the clot is life-saving.

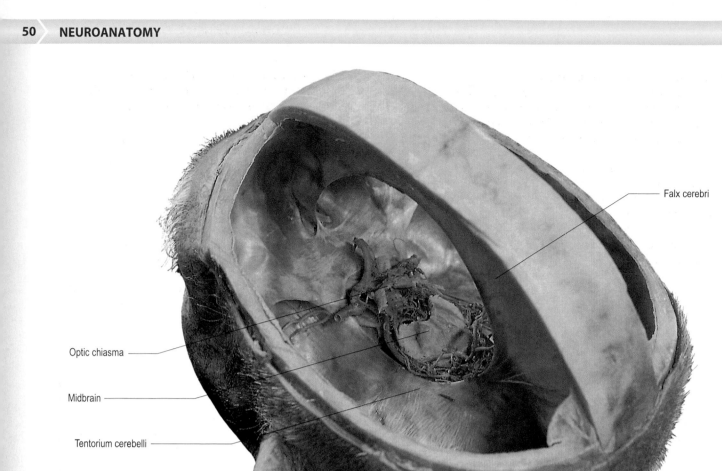

Falx cerebri

Optic chiasma

Midbrain

Tentorium cerebelli

Fig. 5.2 **Cranial cavity showing the arrangement of the dura mater.**

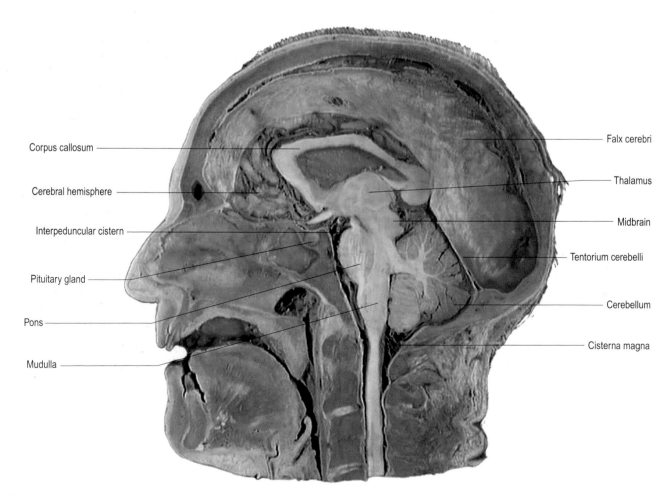

Corpus callosum

Cerebral hemisphere

Interpeduncular cistern

Pituitary gland

Pons

Mudulla

Falx cerebri

Thalamus

Midbrain

Tentorium cerebelli

Cerebellum

Cisterna magna

Fig. 5.3 **Median sagittal section of the head, showing the disposition of the brain and meninges.**

Arachnoid mater and pia mater

The arachnoid mater is a soft, translucent membrane that, like the dura mater, loosely envelops the brain (Figs 1.13 and 6.9). It is separated from the dura by a narrow subdural space, through which pass veins en route to the venous sinuses (Chapter 7).

The pia mater is a microscopically thin, delicate and highly vascular membrane that is closely adherent to the surface of the brain, following all its concavities and convexities. Between the pia and arachnoid mater lies the **subarachnoid space**. This contains a filamentous network of connective tissue strands (trabeculae) and is traversed by numerous arteries and veins. It also contains CSF, which is produced by the choroid plexus within the cerebral ventricles (Chapter 6). Since the arachnoid mater fits loosely round the brain while the pia closely follows its surface contours, the subarachnoid space is of greatly varying depth in different regions. Where significant depressions or fissures in the brain are spanned by the arachnoid mater, **subarachnoid cisterns** are formed. Two of these are particularly large:

- the **cisterna magna**, which lies between the cerebellum and the dorsal surface of the medulla (Figs 5.3 and 5.4). Into this cistern flows CSF from the fourth ventricle.
- the **interpeduncular cistern**, which is located at the base of the brain (Fig. 5.3), where the arachnoid spans the

space between the two temporal lobes. This cistern contains the optic chiasma. The cistern is deepest between the two cerebral peduncles of the midbrain.

Dural venous sinuses

The dura mater is considered to be comprised of two layers. These are normally closely adherent to one another but, in certain locations, become separated to enclose blood-filled spaces, the dural venous sinuses. Major venous sinuses lie in the attached borders of the falx cerebri and tentorium cerebelli and also on the floor of the cranial cavity. Venous blood from the brain flows into these sinuses through a series of interconnecting channels, these in turn drain into the internal jugular vein, through which blood is returned to the general extracranial circulation. The dural venous sinuses are described further in Chapter 7, which deals with the blood supply to the CNS.

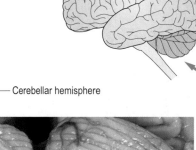

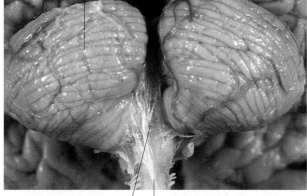

Cerebellar hemisphere

Arachnoid mater
covering cisterna magna

Medulla

Fig. 5.4 **Cisterna magna.**

Cranial meninges

- The dura mater is the outermost membrane. Two dural sheets or reflections extend into the cranial cavity:
  — the falx cerebri, lying between the two cerebral hemispheres
  — the tentorium cerebelli, lying between the cerebellum and the occipital lobes of the cerebrum and encircling the midbrain.
- The dura contains a number of venous sinuses, which are important in the venous drainage of the brain.
- Important sinuses lie within the falx cerebri, tentorium cerebelli and on the floor of the cranial cavity.
- The middle meningeal layer is the arachnoid mater. Both the dura and arachnoid surround the brain loosely.
- The innermost meningeal layer is the pia mater, which adheres to the surface of the brain. This creates a subarachnoid space of variable depth.
- The subarachnoid space contains CSF, which is secreted by the choroid plexus within the cerebral ventricles.

Meningitis

Inflammation of the meninges may result from infection with viruses (e.g. lymphocytic choriomeningitis), bacteria (meningococcal and tuberculous meningitis) or other organisms, or from chemical reaction to injected contrast medium during neuroradiological procedures. The patient complains of headache, photophobia and vomiting, is febrile and has neck stiffness on attempting to move the head. Viral and chemical meningitis are normally mild and self-limiting. Bacterial or fungal meningitis, however, leads to damage to cranial nerves and the brain itself; if untreated, it proceeds to raised intracranial pressure, brain displacement and death.

Chapter 6
Ventricular system and cerebrospinal fluid

The CNS contains an interconnecting series of chambers and channels that are derived from the lumen of the embryonic neural tube. In the spinal cord, this is represented by the vestigial and insignificant central canal. Within the brain, however, the enormous growth and distortion of the basic tube-like structure is paralleled by the development of an elaborate system of ventricles (Figs 6.1 and 6.2).

Topographical anatomy of the ventricular system

In passing from the spinal cord to the brain stem, the central canal moves progressively more dorsal until, in the rostral (open) medulla, it opens out into a wide and shallow depression, the **fourth ventricle** (Fig. 6.3), on the dorsal surface of the brain stem beneath the cerebellum. The fourth ventricle is rhomboid or diamond-shaped. On each side, a **lateral recess** extends towards the lateral margin of the brain stem and is in continuity, through a small **lateral aperture** (the **foramen of Luschka**), with the subarachnoid space of the cerebellopontine angle (Fig. 6.4).

The roof of the rostral part of the fourth ventricle is partly formed by the superior cerebellar peduncles on either side, the space between them being bridged by the thin superior medullary velum. The caudal part of the roof consists of pia and ependyma, a central defect in which constitutes the **median aperture** of the fourth ventricle, or the **foramen of Magendie**, which provides communication with the cisterna magna (Fig. 6.5).

The fourth ventricle extends rostrally as far as the pontomesencephalic junction where it becomes continuous with the **cerebral aqueduct**, which passes throughout the length of the midbrain, beneath the colliculi. At the rostral margin of the midbrain, the cerebral aqueduct opens into the **third ventricle**, which is a narrow slit-like cavity whose lateral walls are formed by the thalamus and hypothalamus on either side (Figs 6.2 and 12.2). The roof of the ventricle is formed by pia–ependyma, which spans between the two striae medullaris thalami, situated along the dorsomedial border of the thalamus. In the rostral part of the third ventricle lies an aperture, the **interventricular foramen** or **foramen of Monro**, which is located between the column of the fornix and the anterior pole of the thalamus.

The interventricular foramen provides communication, on either side, with the extensive **lateral ventricle** located within the cerebral hemisphere (Figs 6.6 and 16.11). The lateral ventricle is approximately C-shaped. It is usually

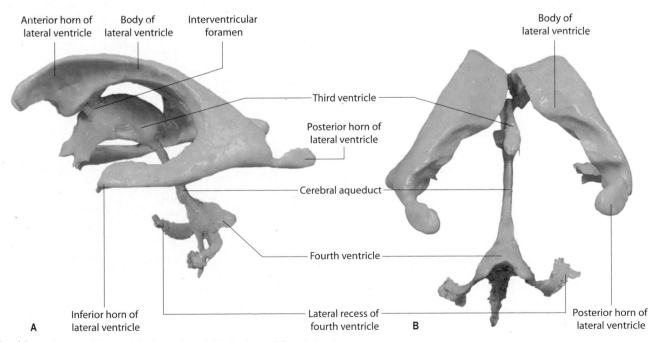

Anterior horn of lateral ventricle   Body of lateral ventricle   Interventricular foramen   Body of lateral ventricle

Third ventricle

Posterior horn of lateral ventricle

Cerebral aqueduct

Fourth ventricle

Inferior horn of lateral ventricle   Lateral recess of fourth ventricle   Posterior horn of lateral ventricle

A   B

Fig. 6.1 **Resin cast of the ventricular system. (A)** Lateral view; **(B)** posterior view.

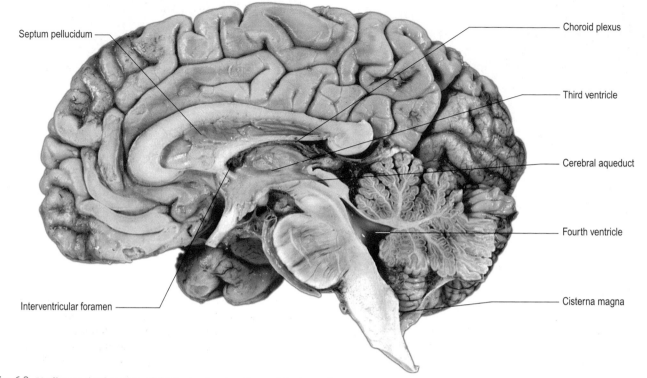

Fig. 6.2 **Median sagittal section of the brain showing the ventricular system.**

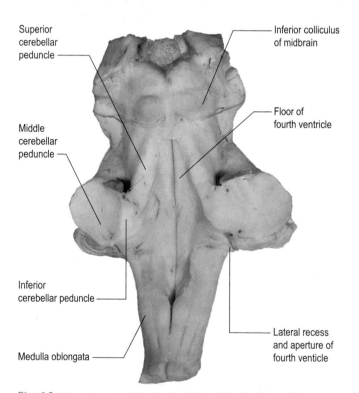

Fig. 6.3 **Dorsal aspect of brain stem illustrating the floor of the fourth ventricle.**

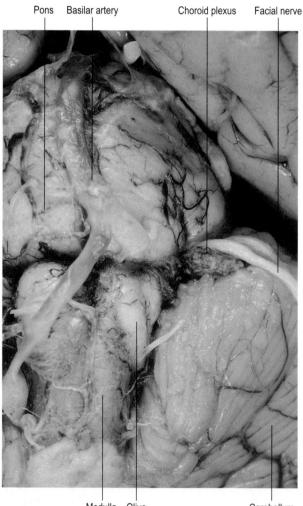

regarded as consisting of an anterior (frontal) horn, body, posterior (occipital) horn and inferior (temporal) horn. The anterior horn of the lateral ventricle is that part anterior to the interventricular foramen. Its lateral wall is the head of the caudate nucleus and its roof is the corpus callosum (Figs 13.3–13.7). The medial wall is formed by the **septum pellucidum**. This thin sheet spans between the corpus callosum and fornix in the midline and separates the

Fig. 6.4 **Cerebellopontine angle.** The point of continuity between the lateral recess of the fourth ventricle and the subarachnoid space is indicated by a small tuft of choroid plexus, which protrudes through the lateral aperture.

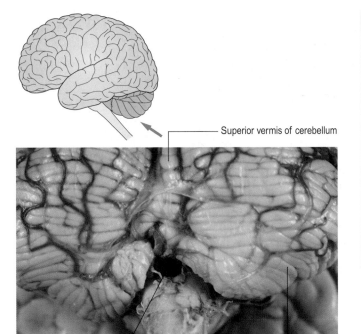

Superior vermis of cerebellum

Median aperture of fourth ventricle

Dorsal aspect of medulla

Cerebellar hemisphere

Fig. 6.5 **Posterior view of the brain.** The cerebellum and brain stem have been slightly separated to show the median aperture of the fourth ventricle.

Topographical anatomy

- The ventricular system consists of lateral, third and fourth ventricles and the cerebral aqueduct.
- The lateral ventricle is located within the cerebral hemisphere and is approximately C-shaped. It communicates, via the interventricular foramen, with the third ventricle.
- The third ventricle is a midline, slit-like cavity. Its lateral walls consist of the thalamus and hypothalamus. Caudally, the third ventricle becomes continuous with the cerebral aqueduct.
- The cerebral aqueduct extends throughout the midbrain, linking the third and fourth ventricles.
- The fourth ventricle is located between the brain stem (pons and medulla) and the cerebellum. A median aperture and two lateral apertures communicate with the subarachnoid space surrounding the brain.

anterior horns of the two lateral ventricles. The body of the lateral ventricle extends behind the interventricular foramen, having as its floor the thalamus and tail of the caudate nucleus. More posteriorly, the small posterior horn extends towards the occipital pole but the principal course of the ventricle sweeps downwards and forwards to form the extensive inferior horn, which lies in the temporal lobe. In the floor of the inferior horn lies the hippocampus, while in its roof runs the much attenuated tail of the caudate nucleus (Figs 13.9–13.12 and 16.11).

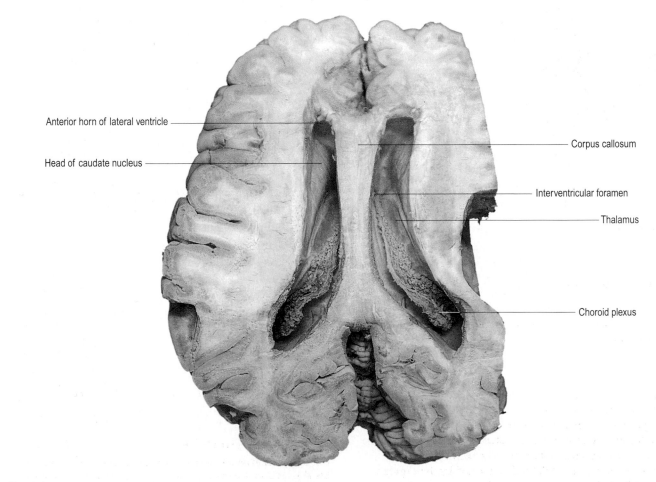

Anterior horn of lateral ventricle

Head of caudate nucleus

Corpus callosum

Interventricular foramen

Thalamus

Choroid plexus

Fig. 6.6 **Superior aspect of a dissection of the cerebral hemispheres in which much of the corpus callosum has been removed to reveal the lumen of the lateral ventricles.**

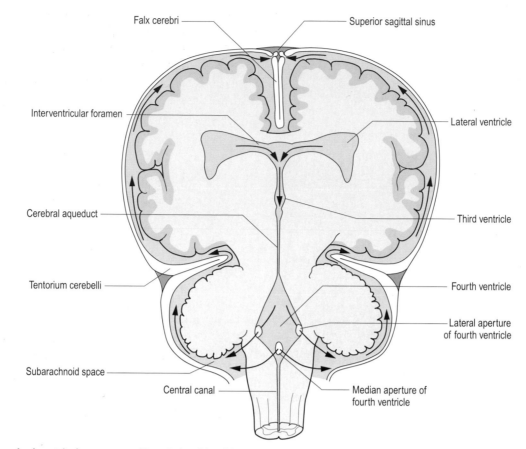

Fig. 6.7 **The cerebral ventricular system and its relationship with the subarachnoid space.** The circulation of cerebrospinal fluid is indicated by arrows.

Cerebrospinal fluid

The ventricular system, together with the cranial and spinal subarachnoid spaces, contains cerebrospinal fluid (CSF). This is produced by the **choroid plexus**, which is located in the lateral, third and fourth ventricles (Figs 6.2, 6.6 and 16.11). The choroid plexus is formed by invagination of the vascular pia mater into the ventricular lumen, where it becomes highly convoluted, producing a sponge-like appearance. The choroid plexus enters the third and fourth ventricles through their roofs and the lateral ventricle through the choroid fissure, along the line of the fimbria/fornix (Figs 16.8 and 16.11).

CSF is produced partly by an active secretory process and partly by passive diffusion. It is a colourless fluid containing little protein and few cells. The volume of CSF in the combined ventricular and subarachnoid spaces is of the order of 150 ml. CSF is produced continuously, at a rate sufficient to fill these spaces several times each day. This means that an efficient mechanism is required for the circulation of CSF and its reabsorption (Figs 6.7 and 6.8).

Most CSF is produced by the choroid plexus of the lateral ventricle. From here it flows through the interventricular foramen into the third ventricle and thence, by way of the cerebral aqueduct, into the fourth ventricle. CSF leaves the ventricular system through the three apertures of the fourth ventricle and, thus, enters the subarachnoid space. Most passes through the median aperture to enter the cisterna magna, located between the medulla and cerebellum. Lesser amounts flow through the lateral apertures to enter the subarachnoid space in the region of the cerebellopontine angle. From these sites, the majority of CSF flows superiorly, round the cerebral hemispheres, to the sites of reabsorption.

Within the subarachnoid space, CSF serves partially to cushion the brain from sudden movements of the head.

CSF is reabsorbed into the venous system by passing into the dural venous sinuses, principally the superior sagittal sinus. Along the sinuses are located numerous **arachnoid villi**, which consist of invaginations of arachnoid mater through the dural wall and into the lumen of the sinus (Fig. 6.8). Reabsorption occurs at these sites because the hydrostatic pressure in the subarachnoid space is higher than that in the sinus lumen and because of the greater colloid osmotic pressure of venous blood compared to CSF. With age, the arachnoid villi become hypertrophic to form **arachnoid granulations** (Fig. 6.9).

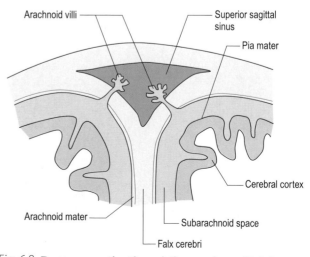

Fig. 6.8 **Transverse section through the superior sagittal sinus showing arachnoid villi.**

Arachnoid granulations

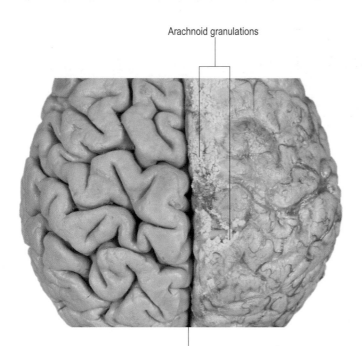

Great longitudinal fissure

Fig. 6.9 **Superior aspect of the cerebral hemispheres showing arachnoid granulations on the right side.** On the left side, the arachnoid mater has been removed.

Hydrocephalus

Obstruction of the flow of CSF within the ventricular system (e.g. by tumours) or the subarachnoid space (e.g. by adhesions following head injury or meningitis) leads to a rise in fluid pressure causing swelling of the ventricles (**hydrocephalus**). The clinical effects are similar to those of a brain tumour and consist of headaches, unsteadiness and mental impairment. Swelling of the optic discs (**papilloedema**) is seen on ophthalmoscopy. Decompression of the dilated ventricles is achieved by inserting a shunt connecting the ventricles to the jugular vein or the abdominal peritoneum.

Cerebrospinal fluid

- Each ventricle contains choroid plexus, which secretes CSF.
- CSF flows in the direction: lateral ventricle → third ventricle → cerebral aqueduct → fourth ventricle → subarachnoid space.
- The combined ventricular system and subarachnoid space contains about 150 ml CSF, this volume being produced several times each day.
- CSF is reabsorbed into the venous system through arachnoid villi, which project into the superior sagittal dural sinus.

Chapter 7
Blood supply of the central nervous system

Blood supply of the spinal cord

Arterial supply of the spinal cord

Three longitudinal vessels run the length of the spinal cord (Fig. 7.1). These are the single **anterior spinal artery** and the paired **posterior spinal arteries**. The anterior spinal artery arises in a Y-shaped configuration from the two vertebral arteries at the level of the medulla (Fig. 7.2) and descends along the ventral surface of the cord in the midline. The posterior spinal arteries arise from either the vertebral arteries or the posterior inferior cerebellar arteries and run caudally on the posterolateral surface of the cord.

The anterior and posterior spinal arteries alone are insufficient to supply the cord below cervical levels and, therefore, they receive serial reinforcement by anastomosis with **radicular arteries** derived from segmental vessels,

> ### Disorders of blood supply of the spinal cord
> The spinal cord and its blood supply are most vulnerable in the thoracic segment and in the anterior portion of the cord. **Occlusion of the anterior spinal artery** leads to an acute thoracic cord syndrome with paraplegia and incontinence. The spinothalamic modalities of pain and temperature are preferentially lost, whereas the proprioceptive functions of the dorsal columns are relatively preserved.

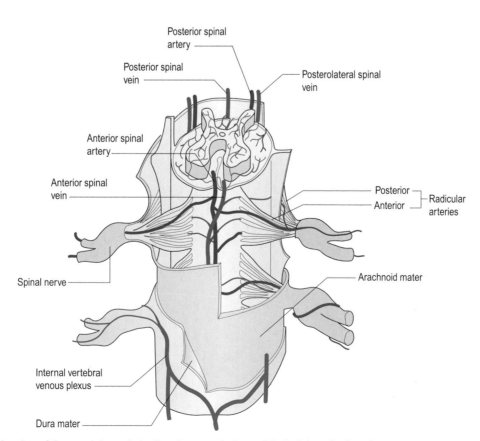

Fig. 7.1 **Schematic drawing of the arterial supply (red) and venous drainage (blue) of the spinal cord.**

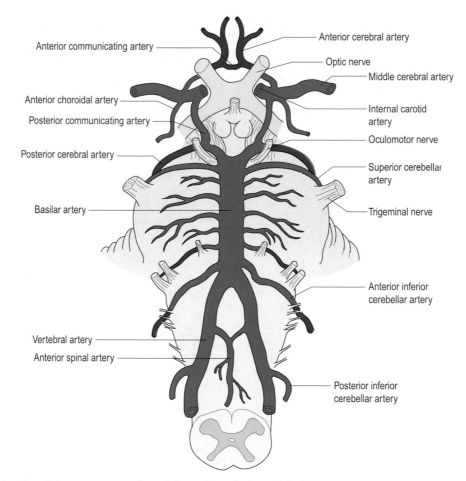

Fig. 7.2 **Schematic drawing of the arrangement of arterial vessels on the base of the brain.** The diagram shows the circulus arteriosus (circle of Willis).

including the ascending cervical, intercostal and lumbar arteries. Radicular arteries pass through the intervertebral foramina and divide into anterior and posterior branches, which run with the dorsal and ventral spinal nerve roots, respectively. One particularly large radicular artery (the **great radicular artery**, or **artery of Adamkiewicz**) may arise from a lateral intercostal or lumbar artery at any level from T8–L3.

Venous drainage of the spinal cord

The venous drainage of the cord follows a basically similar pattern to the arterial supply (Fig. 7.1). Six longitudinal interconnecting venous channels exist. These consist primarily of **anterior** and **posterior spinal veins**, which run in the midline. More irregular, sometimes incomplete, bilaterally paired **anterolateral** and **posterolateral veins** are situated near the lines of attachment of the dorsal and ventral nerve roots. All of these vessels drain via **anterior** and **posterior radicular veins** into the **internal vertebral venous plexus** (epidural venous plexus), which is situated between the dura mater and the vertebral periosteum. The internal venous plexus communicates with an **external**

vertebral venous plexus and hence with the ascending lumbar veins, the azygos and hemiazygos veins.

Blood supply of the brain

Arterial supply of the brain

The brain is supplied with blood by two pairs of vessels, the internal carotid arteries and the vertebral arteries (Figs 7.2 and 7.3). The **internal carotid artery** arises from the common carotid artery and enters the middle fossa of the cranial cavity through the carotid canal. Its course then follows a series of characteristic bends, known as the **carotid syphon** (Fig. 7.5), after which it passes forwards through the cavernous sinus and then upwards on the medial aspect of the anterior clinoid process, reaching the surface of the brain lateral to the optic chiasma. Along its course, the internal carotid artery gives rise to a number of preterminal branches.

- **Hypophyseal arteries** arise from the intracavernous section of the internal carotid to supply the neurohypophysis. They also form the pituitary portal system of vessels by which releasing factors are carried from the hypothalamus to the adenohypophysis.
- The **ophthalmic artery** passes into the orbit through the optic foramen. It supplies the structures of the orbit, the frontal and ethmoidal sinuses, the frontal part of the scalp and dorsum of the nose.
- The **anterior choroidal artery** supplies the optic tract, the choroid plexus of the lateral ventricle, the

---

Blood supply of the spinal cord

- The spinal cord is supplied by the anterior and posterior spinal arteries, supplemented by radicular arteries.
- Venous drainage is by anterior and posterior spinal veins which drain, via radicular veins, into the internal vertebral venous plexus.

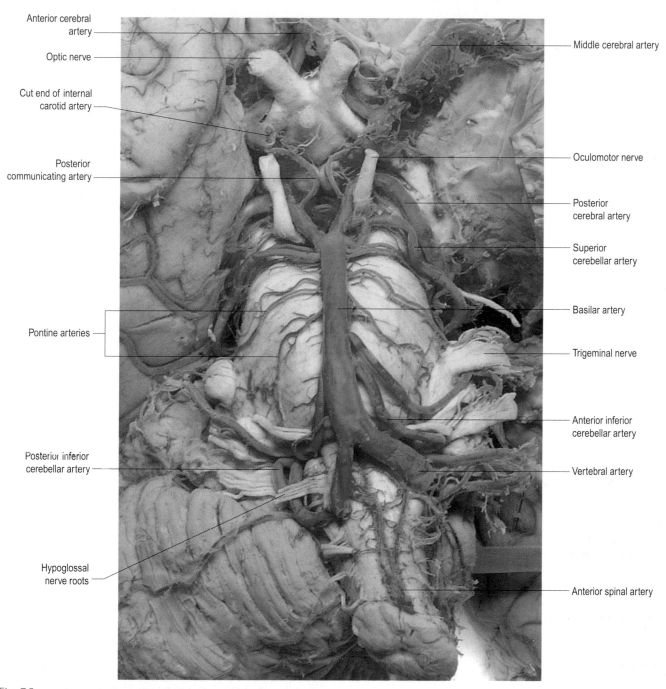

Anterior cerebral artery

Optic nerve

Cut end of internal carotid artery

Posterior communicating artery

Pontine arteries

Posterior inferior cerebellar artery

Hypoglossal nerve roots

Middle cerebral artery

Oculomotor nerve

Posterior cerebral artery

Superior cerebellar artery

Basilar artery

Trigeminal nerve

Anterior inferior cerebellar artery

Vertebral artery

Anterior spinal artery

Fig. 7.3 **Arteries on the base of the brain.** The arterial system has been injected with a red dye.

hippocampus and some of the deep structures of the hemisphere, including the internal capsule and globus pallidus.

■ The **posterior communicating artery** passes backwards to join the posterior cerebral artery, thus forming part of the circle of Willis.

Lateral to the optic chiasma, the internal carotid artery divides into its two terminal branches, the **anterior** and **middle cerebral arteries**. The anterior cerebral artery courses medially above the optic nerve and then passes into the great longitudinal fissure between the frontal lobes. As it does so, it is joined to the corresponding vessel of the opposite side by the short **anterior communicating artery**. Within the great longitudinal fissure, the anterior cerebral artery follows the dorsal curvature of the corpus callosum (Fig. 13.25), branches ramifying over the medial

surface of the frontal and parietal lobes, which it supplies (Fig. 7.4). The territory supplied by the anterior cerebral artery, therefore, includes the motor and sensory cortices for the lower limb. Fine terminal branches also extend out of the great longitudinal fissure to supply a narrow lateral band of frontal and parietal cortices.

The middle cerebral artery is the largest of the three cerebral arteries and its cortical territory is the largest (Fig. 7.4). It passes laterally from its origin to enter the lateral fissure within which it subdivides, branches supplying virtually the whole of the lateral surface of the frontal, parietal and temporal lobes. This includes the primary motor and sensory cortices for the whole of the body, excluding the lower limb. It also serves the auditory cortex and the insula within the depths of the lateral fissure.

Since the structures supplied by branches of the internal carotid artery are normally perfused almost entirely from

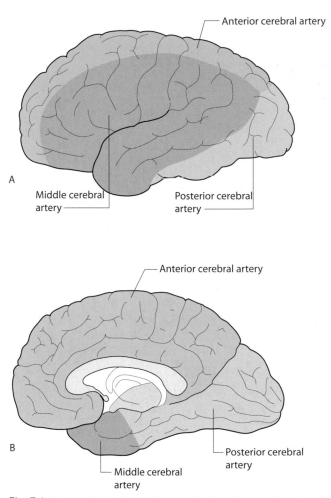

Fig. 7.4 **Schematic drawings of the cerebral hemisphere.** The diagram shows the cortical distribution of the three cerebral arteries. **(A)** Lateral aspect; **(B)** medial aspect.

this source, they are often referred to as being supplied by the 'internal carotid system'.

The **vertebral artery** arises from the subclavian artery, ascends through the foramina transversaria of the cervical vertebrae and enters the cranial cavity through the foramen magnum, alongside the ventrolateral aspect of the medulla (Figs 7.2, 7.3 and 7.6). As they pass rostrally, the two vertebral arteries converge, uniting at the junction between medulla and pons to form the midline **basilar artery**. Along its course, the vertebral artery gives rise to a number of branches, including the anterior and posterior spinal arteries, which supply the medulla and spinal cord. Its largest branch is the **posterior inferior cerebellar artery**, which supplies the inferior aspect of the cerebellum.

The basilar artery runs the length of the pons, which it supplies by means of many small pontine branches. It also gives rise to the **anterior inferior cerebellar artery**, which supplies the anterior and inferior portion of the cerebellum, and the **labyrinthine artery**, which passes into the internal acoustic meatus to supply the inner ear. At the junction of the pons and midbrain, the basilar artery divides into two pairs of vessels, the **superior cerebellar arteries** and the **posterior cerebral arteries**. The superior cerebellar artery supplies the superior aspect of the cerebellum. The posterior cerebral artery curves around the midbrain to supply the visual cortex of the occipital lobe and the inferomedial aspect of the temporal lobe (Fig. 7.4).

The brain regions (brain stem, cerebellum and occipital lobe) served by the vertebral and basilar arteries and their branches are described as being supplied by the 'vertebrobasilar system'.

The internal carotid and vertebrobasilar systems are joined by two thin vessels, the **posterior communicating arteries**, which pass rostrocaudally between the ends of the internal carotid arteries and the posterior cerebral arteries.

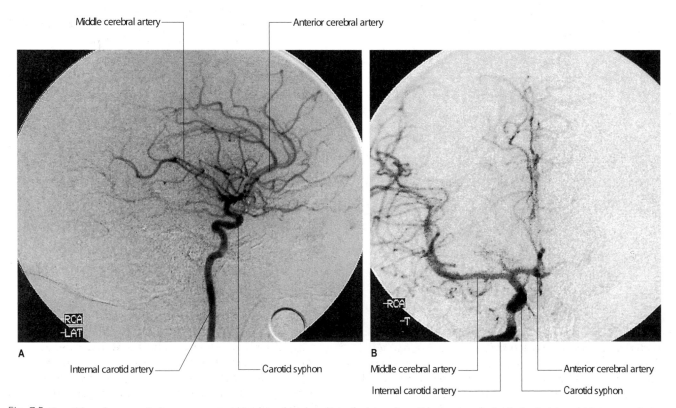

Fig. 7.5 **Carotid angiograms.** Radio-opaque material has been introduced into the internal carotid artery in order to display its intracranial course and distribution. **(A)** Lateral view; **(B)** anteroposterior (Towne's) view. (Courtesy of Professor P D Griffiths)

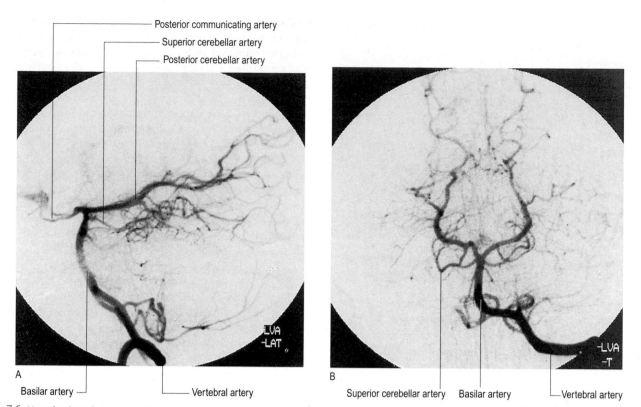

Posterior communicating artery
Superior cerebellar artery
Posterior cerebellar artery

A
Basilar artery — — Vertebral artery

B
Superior cerebellar artery Basilar artery — Vertebral artery

Fig. 7.6 **Vertebral angiograms.** Radio-opaque material has been introduced into the vertebral artery in order to display its intracranial course and distribution. **(A)** Lateral view; **(B)** anteroposterior (Towne's) view. (Courtesy of Professor P D Griffiths)

This completes an anastomosis of vessels on the base of the brain, known as the **circulus arteriosus** or **circle of Willis** (Figs 7.2 and 7.3), which encircles the optic chiasma and the floor of the hypothalamus and midbrain. The anastomotic arrangement of vessels provides the possibility that obstruction or narrowing of the proximal parts of the cerebral arteries, which would be expected to lead to insufficiency in the perfusion of their territories, might be compensated by circulation of blood through the communicating arteries. The actual significance of this arrangement is dependent upon the size of the communicating arteries, which is highly variable between individuals. From the arteries that constitute the circle of Willis, numerous small vessels penetrate the surface of the brain. These are known as the **perforating arteries** (central or ganglionic arteries) and are considered to consist of two groups:

- **anterior perforating arteries**, which arise from the anterior cerebral artery, anterior communicating artery and the region of origin of the middle cerebral artery. They enter the brain in the region between the optic chiasma and the termination of the olfactory tract, known as the anterior perforated substance (Fig. 16.13). These vessels supply large parts of the basal ganglia, the optic chiasma, the internal capsule and hypothalamus.
- **posterior perforating arteries**, which arise from the posterior cerebral and posterior communicating arteries. They enter the brain in the region between the two crura cerebri of the midbrain, known as the posterior perforated substance (Fig. 16.13), to supply the ventral portion of the midbrain and parts of the subthalamus and hypothalamus.

Disorders of blood supply of the brain

One of the most common causes of neurological disability is **stroke**. The sudden occlusion of a cerebral artery leads to death of brain tissue (**infarction**). Rupture of a blood vessel causes bleeding into the brain (**cerebral haemorrhage**). These events lead to the rapid development of a focal neurological syndrome. Strokes related to the carotid artery and its cerebral branches are associated with focal epilepsy, a contralateral sensory/motor deficit and a psychological deficit (e.g. aphasia). Strokes involving the vertebrobasilar circulation lead to a focal brain stem syndrome. Recovery of function can occur but may take up to 2 years and can be incomplete.

An **aneurysm** is an abnormal, balloon-like, swelling of an artery. A surgical emergency arises when an aneurysm ruptures and blood projects around the brain in the subarachnoid space (**subarachnoid haemorrhage**) and into the brain (**intracerebral haemorrhage**). A sudden severe headache and neck stiffness are followed by coma and neurological deficits. Neurosurgery or intra-arterial "coiling" are required to seal the aneurysm to prevent further bleeding and allow recovery.

An **angioma**, or **arteriovenous malformation**, is a congenital collection of swollen blood vessels that can rupture, causing cerebral haemorrhage, or 'steal' blood from adjacent brain regions, leading to epilepsy and a focal cerebral syndrome.

Arterial supply of the brain

- The brain is supplied by paired internal carotid and vertebral arteries.
- The internal carotid artery terminates lateral to the optic chiasma, giving rise to the anterior and middle cerebral arteries.
- The anterior cerebral artery passes into the great longitudinal fissure and supplies the medial aspect of the cerebral hemisphere.
- The middle cerebral artery passes into the lateral fissure and supplies the lateral aspect of the cerebral hemisphere.
- The vertebral arteries run on the ventrolateral aspect of the medulla, uniting to form the midline basilar artery, which extends the length of the pons. Along their course the vertebral and basilar arteries give rise to branches that supply the cerebellum and brain stem.
- The principal terminal branch of the basilar artery is the posterior cerebral artery, which supplies the occipital lobe of the cerebral hemisphere.
- The anterior communicating artery links together the two anterior cerebral arteries. Posterior communicating arteries pass between the internal carotid artery and the posterior cerebral artery, on each side. This anastomosis of vessels constitutes the circle of Willis.
- Small perforating arteries arise from the circle of Willis to supply the hypothalamic area and the internal capsule.

Venous drainage of the brain

Three sets of vessels take part in venous drainage of the brain (Figs 7.7 and 7.8): the superficial veins, the deep veins and the dural venous sinuses. None of these vessels contains valves. **Superficial veins** lie within the subarachnoid space (Fig. 7.7). **Superior cerebral veins** primarily drain the lateral surface of the cerebral hemispheres and empty into the superior sagittal sinus. The **superficial middle cerebral vein** runs along the line of the lateral fissure and empties into the cavernous sinus. In addition, two major anastomotic channels exist, the superior (great) anastomotic vein and the inferior anastomotic vein, which drain into the superior sagittal sinus and the transverse sinus, respectively.

Deep cerebral veins drain the internal structures of the forebrain. Of particular note are the **thalamostriate vein** and the **choroidal vein**, which drain the basal ganglia, thalamus, internal capsule, choroid plexus and hippocampus. These vessels merge to form the **internal cerebral vein**. The two internal cerebral veins then unite in the midline to form the **great cerebral vein** (of Galen), which lies beneath the splenium of the corpus callosum. This short vessel is continuous with the straight sinus, which lies in the midline of the tentorium cerebelli.

The cerebral veins drain into the **dural venous sinuses** (Figs 7.7 and 7.8; see also Chapter 5), which are channels formed between the two layers of dura mater. Major venous sinuses are located in the attached borders of the falx cerebri and the tentorium cerebelli, and on the floor of the cranial cavity.

Along the line where the falx cerebri attaches to the interior of the cranium lies the **superior sagittal sinus**. This receives blood primarily from the superior cerebral veins, which ramify over the lateral surface of the cerebral hemispheres. The free border of the falx encloses the smaller **inferior sagittal sinus**, into which flow veins on the medial aspect of the hemisphere. Within the tentorium cerebelli, along the line of its attachment to the falx, lies the large **straight sinus**. Into this runs the great cerebral vein, which drains the deep structures of the forebrain, and the inferior sagittal sinus.

The superior sagittal sinus and the straight sinus converge at the **confluence of the sinuses**, which lies adjacent to the internal occipital protuberance. From here, blood flows laterally on either side in the **transverse sinus**, which lies along the line of attachment of the tentorium to the occipital bone. The transverse sinus is continuous with the **sigmoid sinus**, which, in turn, joins the **internal jugular vein** at the level of the jugular foramen.

The **cavernous sinus** (Fig. 7.8) lies lateral to the body of the sphenoid bone. It receives blood from the middle cerebral vein and drains into the internal jugular vein (via the inferior petrosal sinus) and into the transverse sinus (via the superior petrosal sinus). The two cavernous sinuses are connected by intercavernous sinuses that lie anterior and posterior to the hypophysis, forming a venous circle around it (the circular sinus). The dural venous sinuses are connected to extracranial veins via **emissary veins**.

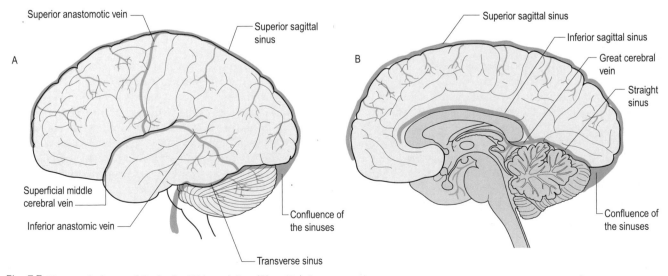

Fig. 7.7 **Venous drainage of the brain. (A)** Lateral view; **(B)** sagittal view.

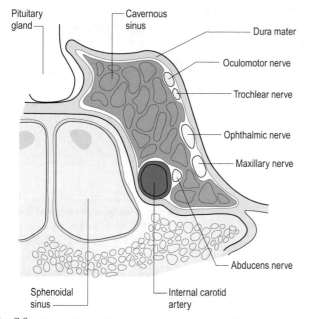

Fig. 7.8 **Schematic drawing of a transverse section through the cavernous sinus.**

 Diseases of the venous sinuses
Thrombosis of the sagittal sinuses is a rare complication of childbirth, blood-clotting disorders and ear infection. Obstruction of the venous drainage of the brain leads to cerebral swelling (**oedema**) and the syndrome of **raised intracranial pressure** (p. 47). Cerebral damage caused by venous infarction manifests as epileptic seizures and focal paralysis of the limbs.

Venous drainage of the brain

- Venous drainage of the brain involves superficial veins, deep veins and dural venous sinuses.
- Superficial veins empty principally into the superior sagittal sinus and the cavernous sinus.
- Deep cerebral veins drain into the great cerebral vein, which is continuous with the straight sinus.
- The superior sagittal sinus and straight sinuses meet at the confluence of the sinuses.
- Venous blood flows, via the transverse sinus and sigmoid sinus, into the internal jugular vein.

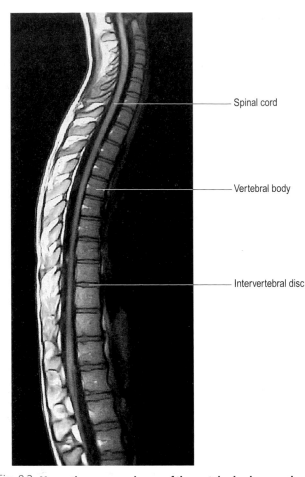

Fig. 8.2 **Magnetic resonance image of the vertebral column and spinal cord in the living subject.** (Courtesy of Professor A Jackson)

Topographical anatomy

- The spinal cord provides sensory, motor and autonomic innervation for the trunk and limbs.
- The cord possesses two enlargements: cervical (C3–T1), associated with innervation of the upper limbs, and lumbar (L1–S3), innervating the lower limbs.
- The cord terminates at vertebral level L1–L2 in the adult.

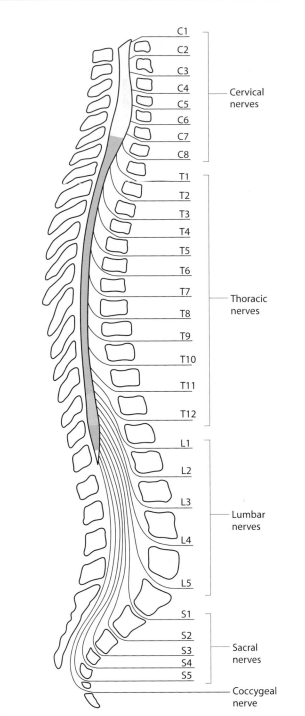

Fig. 8.3 **Schematic representation of the relationships between the spinal cord, spinal nerves and vertebral column.**

elongation of the vertebral column exceeds that of the spinal cord; as a result, at birth the cord terminates at the level of the third lumbar vertebra (L3) and in adult life at the level of the intervertebral disc between L1 and L2 (Figs 8.3 and 8.4).

The approximate level of spinal cord segments may be identified in the living subject by reference to the posterior spinous processes of the vertebrae. As a rule of thumb, cervical cord segments lie approximately one spine higher than their corresponding vertebrae (e.g. C7 cord segment lies adjacent to C6 vertebra), thoracic segments lie approximately two spines higher, and lumbar segments three to four spines higher than their corresponding vertebrae (Fig. 8.3).

Spinal nerves

The spinal cord bears 31 bilaterally paired spinal nerves (8 cervical, 12 thoracic, 5 lumbar, 5 sacral and 1 coccygeal). These originate as two linear series of nerve fascicles attached to the dorsolateral and ventrolateral aspects of the

cord (Fig. 8.5). The groups of six to eight adjacent fascicles that are attached to each cord segment coalesce to form **dorsal** and **ventral nerve roots**. The dorsal and ventral roots of each cord segment then pass to their corresponding **intervertebral foramen** (Fig. 8.6), in or near which they join to form the spinal nerve proper. While the spinal nerves are mixed nerves, containing both afferent and efferent neurones, the dorsal and ventral roots are functionally distinct. The dorsal roots contain **primary afferent neurones** running from peripheral sensory receptors to the spinal cord and brain stem. The nerve cell bodies of these neurones are located in **dorsal root ganglia** (Fig. 8.5), which appear as small enlargements on the dorsal roots near their convergence with the ventral roots at the entrance to the intervertebral foramina. The ventral roots of the spinal

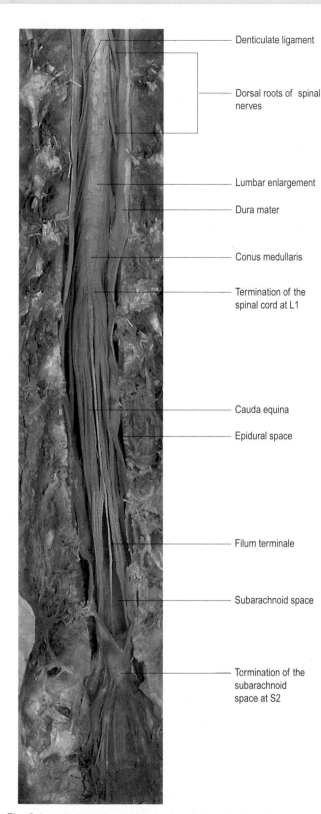

— Denticulate ligament

— Dorsal roots of spinal nerves

— Lumbar enlargement

— Dura mater

— Conus medullaris

— Termination of the spinal cord at L1

— Cauda equina

— Epidural space

— Filum terminale

— Subarachnoid space

— Termination of the subarachnoid space at S2

Fig. 8.4 **Dorsal aspect of the spinal cord caudal to T9–T10.** The dura/arachnoid mater have been cut longitudinally and reflected to reveal the spinal cord and nerve roots within the subarachnoid space.

nerves carry **efferent neurones**, the cell bodies of which are located in the spinal grey matter. These comprise motor neurones, which innervate skeletal muscle, and preganglionic neurones of the autonomic nervous system.

The C1–C7 spinal nerves exit from the vertebral canal above the first seven cervical vertebrae; C8 spinal nerve exits below the seventh cervical vertebra and the remainder leave below their corresponding vertebrae (Fig. 8.3). Because of the

different lengths of the spinal cord and the vertebral canal, only in the cervical region do the spinal cord segments lie adjacent to their corresponding vertebral bodies. Below this level, successive spinal nerve roots follow an increasingly oblique downwards course to reach their respective intervertebral foramina. This is most marked for the lumbar and sacral roots, which descend below the termination of the cord in a leash-like arrangement, the **cauda equina** (Figs 8.3 and 8.4).

Immediately after leaving the intervertebral foramina, spinal nerves divide to produce a thin **dorsal (posterior) ramus** and a much larger **ventral (anterior) ramus** (Figs 8.1 and 8.5). The dorsal ramus supplies the muscles and skin of the back region. The ventral ramus supplies the muscles and skin of the front of the body and the limbs.

The peripheral distribution of spinal nerves, including their pattern of cutaneous innervation (dermatomes) and innervation of muscle groups (myotomes) is described in Chapter 3.

Spinal meninges

The spinal cord, like the brain, is invested by three concentric meningeal coverings: the pia mater, arachnoid mater and dura mater (Figs 8.4 and 8.5).

The innermost covering, the pia mater, is a delicate, vascular membrane that is closely applied to the surface of the cord and nerve roots. Along a line midway between the dorsal and ventral roots of the spinal nerves is attached a

Lumbar puncture and epidural anaesthesia

The lowest part of the spinal canal does not contain the spinal cord; consequently, hollow needles can be safely inserted into the subarachnoid space in order to remove CSF for diagnostic purposes (**lumbar puncture**) or to inject radio-opaque substances for the radiological delineation of the spinal canal and its contents (**myelography**). Similarly, anaesthetics may be introduced into the epidural space in surgical procedures (**epidural block**).

Spinal nerve injury

The spinal nerve roots are vulnerable to compression by degenerative changes in the joints of the spinal column (**spondylosis**) and by **prolapse of intervertebral discs**. Prolapsed intervertebral discs in the cervical spine cause pain in the neck radiating to the arm and hand, accompanied by tingling sensations (paraesthesiae), weakness and wasting of the muscles corresponding to the radicular distribution, and numbness of the skin corresponding to the dermatomal distribution, together with loss of the tendon reflexes subserved by the particular root (Fig. 8.7). Similarly, lumbar prolapsed intervertebral discs lead to back pain and radiation of pain into the legs, known as **sciatica**. A large lumbosacral prolapsed disc may cause paralysis of the bladder and incontinence, demanding urgent neurosurgery.

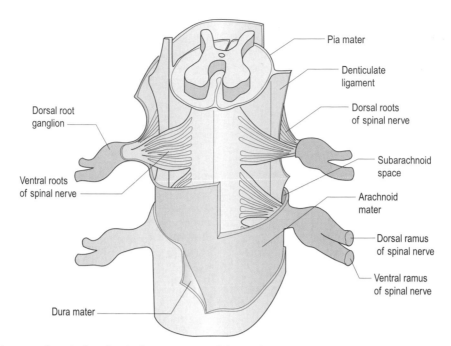

Fig. 8.5 **Relationships between the spinal cord, spinal nerve roots and the meninges.**

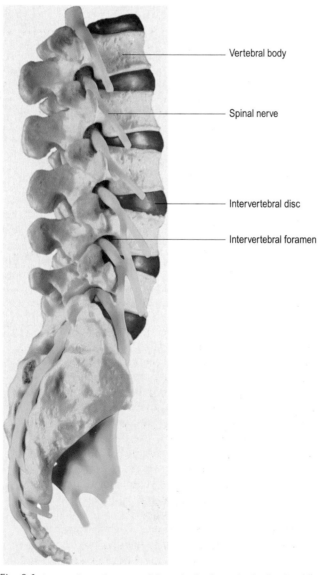

Fig. 8.6 **Posterolateral aspect of the spinal column in the lumbar region illustrating the relationship between the intervertebral foramina and the emerging spinal nerves.**

flat, membranous continuation of the pia, called the **denticulate ligament**. The ligament has a free lateral border for much of its length but, intermittently, lateral projections tether the spinal cord to the arachnoid, and through it to the dura.

The arachnoid mater lies between the pia and dura. It is a translucent membrane that invests the cord like a loose-fitting bag. Between the pia and arachnoid lies the subarachnoid space. This contains CSF, which is produced in the cerebral ventricular system (Chapter 6).

The outer covering of the cord, the dura mater, is a tough, fibrous membrane. It envelops the cord loosely, as does the arachnoid with which it is in contact, though separated by a theoretical plane, the **subdural space**. The dura is separated from the bony wall of the vertebral canal by the **epidural space**.

Although the spinal cord terminates at vertebral level L1–L2, the arachnoid and dural sheaths and, therefore, the subarachnoid space, continue caudally to S2. As the spinal nerve roots pass towards their intervertebral foramina they

Spinal nerves and meninges

- The 31 pairs of spinal nerves attach to the spinal cord as dorsal and ventral roots, carrying afferent and efferent fibres, respectively.
- Spinal nerves exit the vertebral canal via intervertebral foramina.
- Below the termination of the cord, spinal nerve roots descend as the cauda equina.
- The cord and nerve roots are susceptible to traumatic injury, e.g. prolapsed intervertebral disc, cervical spondylosis, spinal dislocation.
- The cord is invested by three meninges (pia, arachnoid and dura mater).
- The subarachnoid space contains CSF.
- CSF may be removed by lumbar puncture at L2–L3 or L3–L4.
- Epidural anaesthesia of lumbar and sacral spinal nerves is possible at the same level.

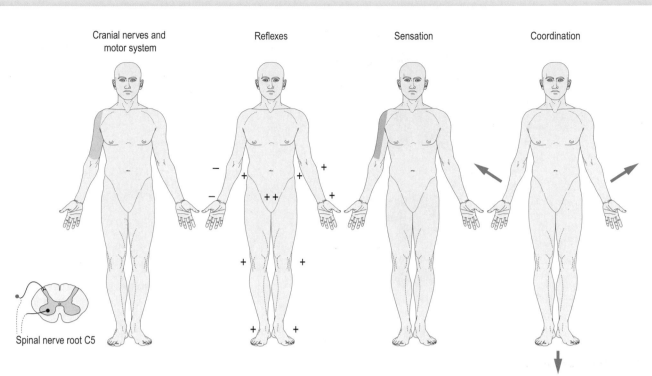

Fig. 8.7 **Spinal nerve root lesion.** For key refer to Figure 1.43.

evaginate the arachnoid and dura, forming meningeal root sleeves that extend as far as the fusion of dorsal and ventral roots. Thereafter, the arachnoid and dura become continuous with the epineurium ensheathing the spinal nerve.

Internal structure of the spinal cord

The spinal cord is incompletely divided into two symmetrical halves by a **dorsal median sulcus** and a **ventral median fissure** (Fig. 8.8). In the centre of the cord is the small **central canal**, which is continuous rostrally with the cerebral ventricular system. Surrounding the central canal is the spinal **grey matter**, consisting of nerve cell bodies, their dendrites and synaptic contacts. The outer part of the cord consists of **white matter**, which contains

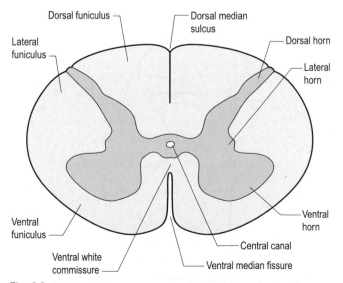

Fig. 8.8 **Schematic transverse section through the spinal cord showing the general disposition of grey and white matter.**

Motor neuronopathies

The lower motor neurones of the spinal cord may be selectively affected by two diseases.

Poliomyelitis is an acute viral infection of the neurones leading to rapid paralysis and wasting of the limb and respiratory muscles. The disability is often asymmetrical and frequently affects the legs. Recovery occurs but may be incomplete.

Motor neurone disease is a chronic degenerative disorder that affects both lower motor neurones and the descending tracts to the spinal cord (upper motor neurones). Degeneration of ventral horn cells causes weakness, wasting, hypotonia and fasciculation of the limb muscles (**progressive muscular atrophy**). Degeneration of descending pathways leads to weakness and spasticity of the limb muscles (**amyotrophic lateral sclerosis**).

ascending and descending nerve fibres. Some serve to join neighbouring and distant cord segments for the integration of their functions, while others run between the cord and the brain. Many of the fibres that share a common origin, course and termination are grouped together in fascicles, forming the long **tracts** of the spinal cord.

Different cord levels vary in the relative amounts and configuration of grey and white matter (Fig. 8.9). Higher levels contain greater amounts of white matter. This is because ascending tracts gain fibres at each successive level, whereas the opposite is true of descending tracts.

Grey matter of the spinal cord

The grey matter is approximately H-shaped, or butterfly-shaped, with four protrusions, the **dorsal (posterior)** and **ventral (anterior) horns**, extending dorso- and ventrolaterally towards the attachment zones of the dorsal and ventral root fascicles, respectively. The size and shape of

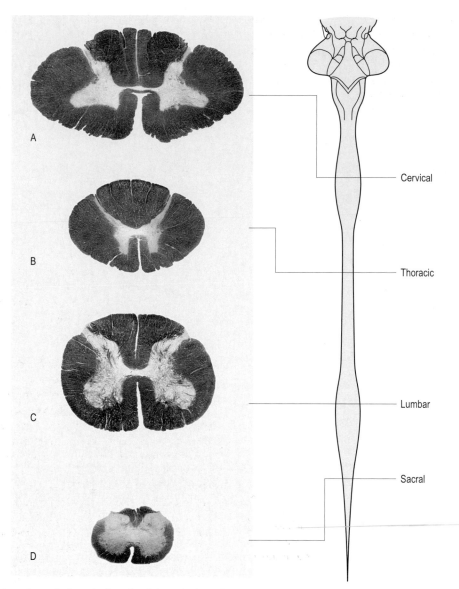

Fig. 8.9 **Transverse sections through the spinal cord at (A) cervical, (B) thoracic, (C) lumbar and (D) sacral levels.** The histological method employed (Weigert–Pal) stains white matter (myelinated nerve fibres), leaving grey matter (nerve cell bodies) relatively unstained.

the dorsal and ventral horns varies according to the level (Fig. 8.9). Many afferent nerve fibres entering in the dorsal roots terminate in the dorsal horn, while the ventral horn contains the cell bodies of motor neurones that exit through the ventral nerve roots and innervate skeletal muscle. Both dorsal and ventral horns are, therefore, particularly well developed at cervical and lumbar levels in association with innervation of the upper and lower limbs. Thoracic and upper lumbar segments additionally possess a small **lateral** or **intermediolateral horn**, located between the dorsal and ventral horns, which contains the cell bodies of **preganglionic sympathetic neurones** (Figs 8.8 and 8.9).

The grey matter of the spinal cord may be divided, on the basis of its cytoarchitecture, into ten zones, known as **Rexed's laminae**, which are numbered sequentially from dorsal to ventral (Fig. 8.10). Some of these laminae are equated with cell groupings of particular functional types.

Dorsal horn

Afferent fibres entering through the dorsal roots divide into ascending and descending branches. They mostly terminate

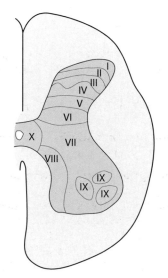

Fig. 8.10 **Lamination of spinal grey matter (Rexed's laminae).**

near their point of entry but may travel for varying distances in either direction, running in the **dorsolateral fasciculus** or **Lissauer's tract**, which is located superficial to the tip of the dorsal horn (see Fig. 8.14). Dorsal root afferents may, therefore, establish synaptic contacts over several segments of spinal grey matter. Dorsal root fibres terminate extensively within the grey matter but most densely in the dorsal horn. Cutaneous afferents tend to terminate in superficial (dorsal) laminae, while proprioceptive and muscle afferents project mostly to deeper laminae.

The tip of the dorsal horn, approximating to Rexed's laminae I–III, is also known as the **substantia gelatinosa**. This region receives collaterals of the smallest-diameter myelinated (group A delta) and unmyelinated (group C) afferents that are associated with nociception. These neurones are excitatory and use glutamic acid and the peptide substance P as neurotransmitters. In the substantia gelatinosa, complex interactions occur with other types of afferent terminal, interneurones, and with descending pathways from the brain, which control the transmission of pain information to ascending spinothalamic and spinoreticular tract neurones distributed throughout the dorsal horn. For example, input from large-diameter afferents carrying tactile information is thought to inhibit transmission of nociceptive impulses to ascending tract neurones, which may explain why rubbing a sore spot can relieve pain.

The substantia gelatinosa contains high levels of the endogenous opioid peptide enkephalin, which is thought to act as a transmitter of some dorsal horn interneurones. These establish presynaptic contacts with the terminals of primary afferent neurones that possess opiate receptors. Occupation of these receptors decreases the release of substance P. The analgesic properties of opiates such as morphine are partly a result of their action at this site.

Deeper in the dorsal horn, lamina VII contains a number of important cell groups. At cord levels C8–L3 lie the cells of **Clarke's column** (thoracic nucleus, nucleus dorsalis), which are the origin of ascending fibres of the dorsal spinocerebellar tract. The cells of Clarke's column receive afferent input from muscle spindles, Golgi tendon organs, tactile and pressure receptors. At thoracic and upper lumbar levels, the lateral part of lamina VII also contains preganglionic sympathetic neurones that constitute the lateral horn, while at sacral levels (S2–S4) it contains preganglionic parasympathetic neurones.

Ventral horn

In the ventral horn, lamina IX corresponds to groups of motor neurones that innervate skeletal muscle. These are of two types:

- **alpha motor neurones**, which innervate extrafusal muscle fibres
- **gamma motor neurones**, which innervate intrafusal muscle fibres (within muscle spindles).

The ventral horn is particularly well developed in the cervical and lumbar enlargements owing to the presence of motor neurones innervating the upper and lower limbs. Generally speaking, neurones innervating axial musculature (neck and trunk) tend to be located medially, while those innervating limb muscles are positioned more laterally. In the ventral horn of cord segments C3–C5 is located the **phrenic nucleus**, a group of motor neurones that innervate the

---

> ## Grey matter of the spinal cord
>
> - Internally, the spinal cord consists of a central core of grey matter (cell bodies) and an outer mantle of white matter (nerve fibres).
> - Within the grey matter, the dorsal horn is the main site of termination of primary afferent fibres. It includes the substantia gelatinosa, which is important in transmission of nociceptive impulses to the brain.
> - The lateral horn contains preganglionic sympathetic neurones.
> - The ventral horn contains alpha and gamma motor neurones, also known as lower motor neurones.

diaphragm via the phrenic nerve and are, thus, essential for breathing. Cells in the ventral horn receive direct input from certain dorsal root afferents (e.g. from muscle spindles for mediation of the stretch reflex). Importantly, they also receive input from pathways descending from higher centres concerned with motor control.

Spinal reflexes

A reflex is an involuntary, stereotyped pattern of response brought about by a sensory stimulus. Although the qualitative nature of an established reflex response is constant, it may vary considerably in a quantitative sense (e.g. in delay, duration and extent) as a result of intersegmental and supraspinal influences.

Anatomically, the pathways mediating reflex actions consist of afferent neurones conveying impulses from sensory receptors to the CNS (spinal cord or brain stem) and efferent neurones running from the CNS to the effector organ (muscle or gland). In all but the simplest reflexes, interneurones within the CNS are interposed between the afferent and efferent components. The internal organisation of the spinal cord (and brain stem) thus subserves a number of more or less complex reflex functions, some of which are both relatively well understood and clinically important.

Stretch reflex

If a muscle is stretched, it responds by contracting, and this is known as the **stretch** or **myotatic reflex**. Anatomically, this is the simplest of reflexes and is mediated by a **monosynaptic reflex arc** (Fig. 8.11). It consists of afferent neurones that convey impulses from muscle stretch receptors to the CNS and motor neurones that convey impulses back to the stretched muscle.

Stretch receptors within muscles consist of sensory nerve endings that attach to the central, non-contractile region of specialised muscle cells called **intrafusal muscle fibres**. Intrafusal muscle fibres are oriented parallel to the long axis of the main muscle and occur in groups called **muscle spindles**. Stretch applied to the muscle in which they lie stimulates the sensory endings. Their afferent fibres carry impulses to the CNS, where they make monosynaptic excitatory contact with alpha motor neurones that innervate the bulk of the muscle (**extrafusal muscle fibres**) and make it contract.

There are two types of intrafusal muscle fibre: **nuclear bag** and **nuclear chain** fibres. These bear two types of sensory ending:

- the **primary** or **annulospiral ending**, associated with group Ia afferent fibres,

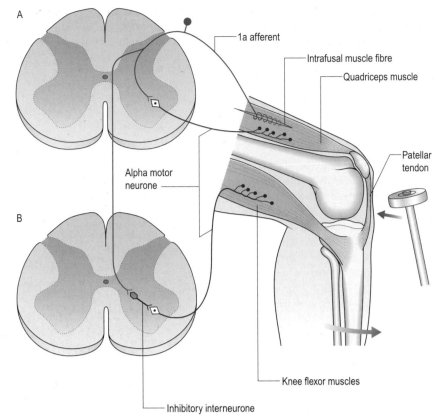

Fig. 8.11 **The stretch reflex and reciprocal innervation. (A)** The quadriceps stretch reflex is illustrated, whereby striking the patellar tendon elicits extension of the knee; **(B)** Reciprocal innervation. While stretching of the quadriceps muscle causes its reflex contraction, the motor neurones of antagonistic muscles (knee flexors) are inhibited by interneuronal connection within the spinal cord.

- the **secondary** or **flower-spray ending**, associated with group II afferents.

When a muscle is stretched, these endings are stimulated. Primary endings have both velocity and length sensitivity, while secondary endings have essentially only length sensitivity. Group Ia afferents from a particular muscle make excitatory monosynaptic contact with alpha motor neurones innervating the same muscle and, thus, mediate the myotatic reflex.

Stretch reflexes are important in the control of skeletal muscle tone, which refers to the degree of resistance to passive movement and is determined by the proportion of motor units that are active at any one time. When the upper motor neurones are damaged, muscle tone is increased during initial muscle stretch (spasticity). Since stretch reflexes operate to maintain muscles at a constant length in opposition to imposed stretch, they are important in the control of posture. By their action activity is maintained in neck, trunk and lower limb extensor muscles (anti-gravity muscles) that support an upright body posture against the force of gravity and are stretched when these body parts become flexed.

In addition to alpha motor neurones, which innervate extrafusal muscle fibres, the ventral horn of the spinal cord (and motor cranial nerve nuclei) contain **gamma motor neurones**, which innervate the polar, contractile elements of intrafusal muscle fibres (Fig. 8.12). When gamma motor neurones are activated, the resultant contraction of the intrafusal muscle fibre applies tension to the sensory

Tendon reflexes

Deep tendon reflexes, or tendon jerks, are monosynaptic stretch reflexes elicited during clinical examination by percussion of the tendon of the muscle by a tendon hammer. Each tendon reflex is subserved by certain spinal cord segments:

Reflex	Cord segments
Biceps reflex (biceps jerk)	C5/C6
Brachioradialis reflex (supinator jerk)	C5/C6
Triceps reflex (triceps jerk)	C6/C7
Quadriceps reflex (knee jerk)	L3/L4
Achilles tendon reflex (ankle jerk)	S1/S2

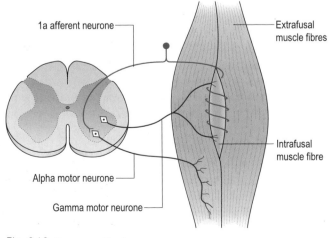

Fig. 8.12 **Gamma reflex loop.**

endings. This lowers the threshold of the stretch receptors to externally applied stretch and, thus, increases the sensitivity of the stretch reflex (the **gamma reflex loop**, Fig. 8.12).

Like alpha motor neurones, gamma motor neurones are under the influence of descending pathways from the brain. Abnormalities in the activity of these pathways, therefore, which occur in many pathological conditions, induce changes in the sensitivity of stretch reflexes. This is evidenced by abnormalities in muscle tone.

When a stretch reflex is elicited (e.g. the quadriceps reflex, by tapping the patellar tendon), primary afferent fibres from the muscle spindle excite not only the alpha motor neurones of the stretched muscle but also interneurones that inhibit the alpha motor neurones of antagonistic muscles (e.g. the knee flexors, Fig. 8.11). This illustrates the general principle of **reciprocal innervation** of agonist and antagonist muscle groups.

Flexor reflex

Noxious cutaneous stimulation of the limbs causes withdrawal from the offending stimulus. This is mediated by a **polysynaptic reflex** in which one or more interneurones are interposed between afferent and efferent neurones. Primary afferent fibres activate interneurones within the spinal grey matter, which in turn excite alpha motor neurones innervating the limb flexor muscles (Fig. 8.13). Flexion of a limb about several joints requires the coordinated action of more than one spinal segment and this is achieved by collateralisation of primary afferents and interneurones.

All forms of cutaneous stimulation have the potential to elicit the flexor reflex, but this is normally prevented by descending pathways from the brain unless the stimulus is painful. In certain pathological conditions, the descending inhibitory influence is lost and even innocuous cutaneous stimulation can cause limb withdrawal. The extensor plantar (Babinski) response is a partial flexion withdrawal of the great toe on stimulation of the sole of the foot.

Activation of the flexor reflex in a weight-bearing limb (e.g. by standing on a pin) simultaneously causes reflex extension of the contralateral limb to take the weight of the body. This is called the **crossed extensor reflex** (Fig. 8.13). It is mediated by axon collaterals which cross the midline of the cord and excite the alpha motor neurones of contralateral limb extensor muscles.

Spinal reflexes

- The internal organisation of the cord subserves a number of important reflex functions.
- The monosynaptic stretch reflex mediates muscle contraction in response to stretch of muscle spindles.
- The sensitivity of the stretch reflex is regulated by gamma motor neurones, which provide motor innervation to the spindle fibres.
- The stretch reflex is responsible for maintenance of muscle tone and is clinically tested as the deep tendon reflexes.

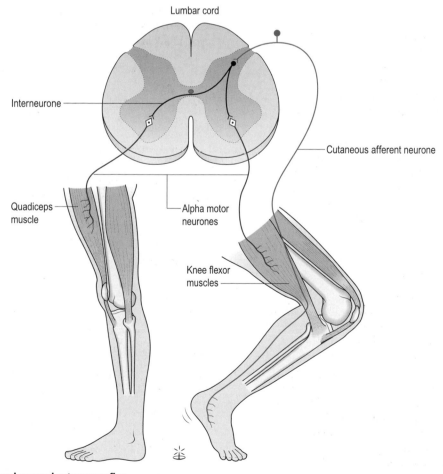

Lumbar cord

Interneurone

Cutaneous afferent neurone

Quadiceps muscle

Alpha motor neurones

Knee flexor muscles

Fig. 8.13 **Flexor reflex and crossed extensor reflex.**

White matter of the spinal cord

The grey matter of the spinal cord is completely surrounded by white matter, which consists of ascending and descending nerve fibres. The white matter is sometimes considered to be divided into dorsal, lateral and ventral columns or **funiculi** (Fig. 8.8). Nerve fibres sharing common origins, terminations and functions are organised into **tracts** or **fasciculi** (Latin: small bundles). Some fibres interconnect adjacent or distant cord segments and permit intersegmental coordination, while other fibres are longer and serve to join the spinal cord with the brain. The **intersegmental**, or **propriospinal**, fibres occupy a narrow band immediately peripheral to the grey matter. This is known as the **fasciculus proprius** (Fig. 8.14). Nerve fibres running between the spinal cord and the brain constitute the **ascending** and **descending tracts** of the spinal cord (Figs 8.14–8.20).

Ascending spinal tracts

Ascending tracts carry impulses from pain, thermal, tactile, muscle and joint receptors to the brain. Some of this information eventually reaches a conscious level (the cerebral cortex), while some is destined for subconscious centres (e.g. the cerebellum).

Pathways that carry information to a conscious level share certain common characteristics.

There is a sequence of three neurones between the peripheral receptor and the cerebral cortex.

- The first neurone (first-order neurone or primary afferent neurone) enters the spinal cord through the dorsal root of a spinal nerve and its cell body lies in the dorsal root ganglion. The central process may collateralise extensively and make synaptic connections that mediate spinal reflexes and intersegmental coordination. The main fibre remains on the ipsilateral side of the cord and terminates in synaptic contact with the second neurone either in the spinal grey matter or in the medulla oblongata of the brain stem.

- The second neurone (second-order neurone) has its cell body in the cord or medulla oblongata. Its axon crosses over (decussates) to the opposite side of the CNS and ascends to the thalamus, where it terminates upon the third neurone.

- The third-order neurone has its cell body in the thalamus. Its axon passes to the somatosensory cortex of the parietal lobe of the cerebral hemisphere.

Two main tract systems in the spinal cord fit into this pattern: the dorsal (posterior) columns and the spinothalamic tracts.

Dorsal columns

The dorsal columns are located between the dorsal median sulcus and the dorsal horn. Two tracts are recognised:

- the **fasciculus gracilis**, situated medially
- the **fasciculus cuneatus**, situated laterally.

The tracts carry impulses concerned with proprioception (movement and joint position sense) and discriminative touch.

The dorsal columns contain the axons of primary afferent neurones that have entered the cord through the dorsal roots of spinal nerves (Fig. 8.15). The fasciculus gracilis consists of fibres that join the cord at sacral, lumbar and lower thoracic levels; fibres of the fasciculus cuneatus enter

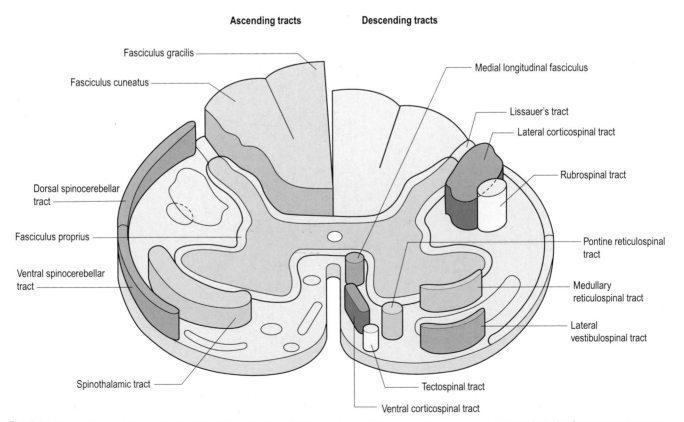

Fig. 8.14 **Ascending and descending tracts of the spinal cord.** All ascending and descending tracts are present bilaterally. In this figure, ascending tracts are emphasised on the left side and descending tracts are emphasised on the right side. In addition, the location of Lissauer's tract and the fasciculus proprius (which contain both ascending and descending fibres) are shown.

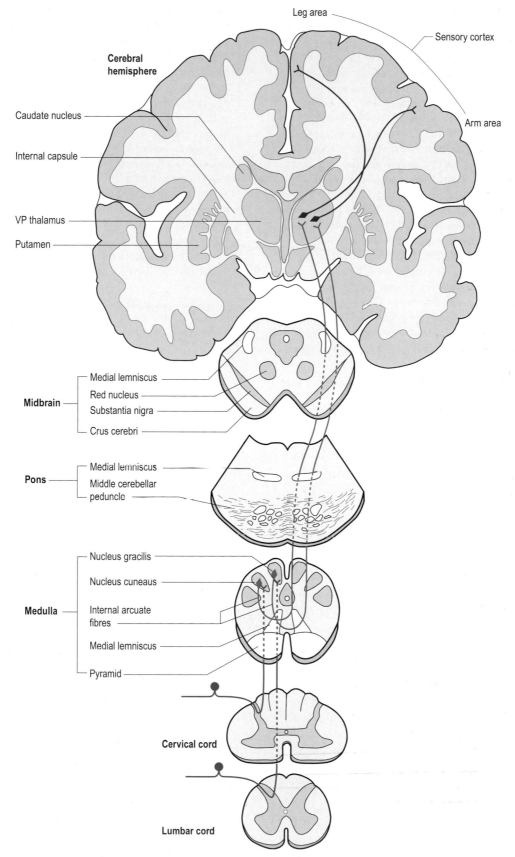

Fig. 8.15 **The dorsal column system.** The central pathways carrying conscious proprioception and discriminative touch are illustrated.

via the upper thoracic and cervical dorsal roots. Since the dorsal columns contain primary afferent neurones, they carry information relating to the ipsilateral side of the body. Fibres ascend without interruption to the medulla oblongata where they terminate upon second-order neurones, the cell

bodies of which are located in the **nucleus gracilis** and **nucleus cuneatus**.

The axons of second-order neurones decussate in the medulla as **internal arcuate fibres** and, thereafter, ascend through the brain stem as the **medial lemniscus**. The

Lesions of the dorsal columns

Tabes dorsalis is a late manifestation of syphilitic infection of the CNS. It chiefly affects the lumbosacral dorsal spinal roots and the dorsal columns of the spinal cord. The loss of proprioception leads to a high steppage and unsteady gait (**sensory ataxia**), which is exacerbated when the eyes are closed (**Romberg's sign**).

Subacute combined degeneration of the spinal cord is a systemic disease resulting from a deficiency of vitamin B_{12} (cyanocobalamin), which also causes pernicious anaemia. The degeneration of the dorsal columns produces sensory ataxia. The lateral columns of the spinal cord are also involved (combined), causing weakness and spasticity of the limbs. The disorder, although uncommon, is an important one since proper treatment with vitamin B_{12} can lead to complete recovery.

In **multiple sclerosis**, an immune disease, specific damage to the fasciculus cuneatus of the cervical spinal cord leads to loss of proprioception in the hands and fingers, causing profound loss of dexterity and inability to identify the shape and nature of objects by touch alone (**astereognosis**).

Spinothalamic tract lesions

The spinothalamic tracts can be selectively damaged in **syringomyelia**, in which the central canal becomes enlarged to form a cavity compressing adjacent nerve fibres. The second-order neurones subserving pain and temperature are damaged as they decussate in the ventral white commissure, close to the central canal, causing a selective loss of pain and temperature awareness in the upper limbs. This is termed a **dissociated sensory loss**, since light touch and proprioceptive sensation are retained. The patient injures and burns the hands painlessly, and joints of the limbs become disorganised without discomfort (**Charcot's joints**).

Selective surgical destruction of the spinothalamic tracts (**cordotomy** or **tractotomy**) is sometimes performed for the neurosurgical relief of intractable pain from a variety of causes.

medial lemniscus terminates in the **ventral posterior (VP) nucleus** of the thalamus upon third-order thalamocortical neurones, which project to the somatosensory cortex.

Spinothalamic tract

The spinothalamic tract lies lateral and ventral to the ventral horn of the spinal grey matter. It carries information related to pain and thermal sensations and also non-discriminative touch and pressure. Some authorities identify distinct lateral and ventral spinothalamic tracts conveying pain and temperature or touch and pressure, respectively, but fibres carrying these modalities are probably intermingled, at least to some extent.

The spinothalamic tract contains second-order neurones, the cell bodies of which lie in the contralateral dorsal horn and receive input from primary afferent fibres that terminate in this region (Fig. 8.16). After leaving the parent cell bodies, spinothalamic axons decussate to the opposite side of the cord by passing through the **ventral white commissure**, which lies ventral to the central canal of the cord, and, thus, enter the contralateral spinothalamic tract. Axons carrying pain and temperature decussate within one segment of their origin, while those carrying touch and pressure may ascend for several segments before crossing.

In the brain stem, the spinothalamic fibres run in proximity to the medial lemniscus and are known as the **spinal lemniscus**. The majority of fibres terminate in the ventral posterior nucleus of the thalamus, contacting third-order thalamocortical neurones that project to the somatosensory cortex.

The spinothalamic tract is sometimes referred to as the neospinothalamic system. It is highly organised somatotopically; consequently, the origin of sensory stimuli can be accurately localised. It is thought to be the route via which sharp, pricking pain (sometimes called 'fast' pain) is conducted.

The **spinoreticulothalamic system** represents an additional, phylogenetically older, route by which sensory impulses ascend to higher centres. Some second-order neurones arising from the dorsal horn ascend in the ventrolateral region of the cord and then terminate in the brain stem reticular formation, particularly within the medulla. Reticulothalamic fibres then ascend to the intralaminar thalamic nuclei, which in turn activate the cerebral cortex. The spinoreticulothalamic system is thought to be the route via which dull, aching pain (sometimes called 'slow' pain) is transmitted to a conscious level. Activation of spinothalamic and spinoreticular fibres, which may ultimately be perceived as unpleasant or painful, can be modulated by descending pathways from the brain.

Ascending pathways that carry impulses to a subconscious level are represented by the spinocerebellar tracts.

Spinocerebellar tracts

Fibres of the ascending spinocerebellar tracts form dorsal and ventral tracts that are located near the dorsolateral and ventrolateral surfaces of the cord, respectively. Both tracts carry information derived from muscle spindles, Golgi tendon organs and tactile receptors to the cerebellum for the control of posture and coordination of movement.

The spinocerebellar system consists of a sequence of only two neurones. Both spinocerebellar tracts contain second-order neurones whose cell bodies of origin lie in the base of the dorsal horn; they receive input from primary afferent

Friedreich's ataxia

Friedreich's ataxia is an inherited degenerative disease in which the spinocerebellar tracts are particularly disordered, leading to profound incoordination of the arms (intention tremor) and a wide-based, reeling gait (ataxia). The disorder begins in childhood and the patient is wheelchair-bound by 20 years of age.

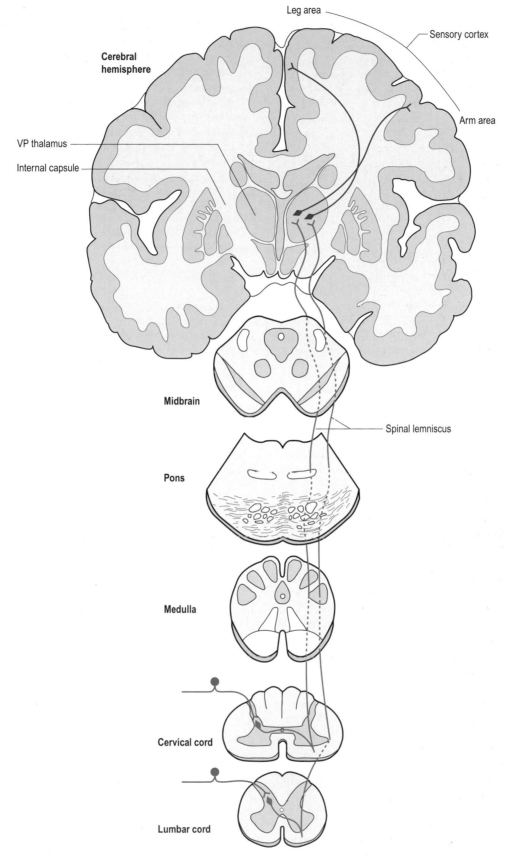

Fig. 8.16 **The spinothalamic tract system.** The central pathways for pain, temperature, touch and pressure are illustrated.

fibres terminating in this region. The tract neurones terminate directly in the cerebellar cortex, predominantly within the vermis. Fibres of the dorsal spinocerebellar tract originate from a prominent group of cells known as **Clarke's column**. The axons ascend ipsilaterally to enter

the cerebellum through the **inferior cerebellar peduncle**. Fibres of the ventral spinocerebellar tract decussate, ascend on the contralateral side of the cord and enter the cerebellum via the **superior cerebellar peduncle**. Some axons then recross within the cerebellar white matter.

White matter of the spinal cord: principal ascending tracts

Ascending tracts carry afferent information to conscious and subconscious levels. Pathways to a conscious level follow a basic plan of three neurones in a chain from peripheral receptor to cerebral cortex.

Dorsal columns (fasciculus gracilis and cuneatus) carry proprioception and discriminative touch. They convey first-order neurones ipsilaterally to the nuclei gracilis and cuneatus of the medulla. Second-order neurones decussate and pass to the thalamus. Third-order neurones project to the somatosensory cortex. Lesions (e.g. tabes dorsalis, vitamin B_{12} deficiency) lead to ataxia and loss of discriminative touch.

Spinothalamic tracts carry pain, temperature, touch and pressure. The tract contains second-order neurones with cell bodies in the dorsal horn. Axons decussate and pass to the thalamus. Third-order neurones project to the somatosensory cortex. Lesions (e.g. syringomyelia) lead to impairment of pain, temperature, touch and pressure sensitivity on the contralateral side.

Dorsal and ventral spinocerebellar tracts contain second-order neurones carrying muscle, joint and tactile information involved in motor control. Lesions lead to ataxia (e.g. Friedreich's ataxia).

Hereditary spastic paraparesis

Hereditary spastic paraparesis is an inherited degenerative disorder (autosomal dominant) in which progressive weakness affects the legs, leading to marked stiffness of gait. Degeneration of the lateral columns, including the lateral corticospinal tract, chiefly affects the thoracic spinal cord, causing a spastic paraparesis with hyperreflexia and extensor plantar responses, but with sparing of sensation and bladder function.

Descending spinal tracts

Descending tracts of the spinal cord (Fig. 8.14) originate from the cerebral cortex and brain stem. They are concerned with the control of movement, muscle tone, spinal reflexes, spinal autonomic functions and the modulation of sensory transmission to higher centres.

Corticospinal tracts

The corticospinal tracts (Fig. 8.17) are particularly concerned with the control of voluntary, discrete, skilled movements, especially those of the distal parts of the limbs. Such movements are sometimes referred to as 'fractionated' movements. Corticospinal tract neurones arise from cell bodies in the cerebral cortex. The cells of origin are widely distributed in the motor and sensory cortices, including the **precentral gyrus** or **primary motor cortex**, where the large **Betz cells** give rise to the largest diameter corticospinal axons. Corticospinal axons leave the cerebral hemispheres by passing through the massive subcortical fibre systems of the **corona radiata** and **internal capsule** to enter the **crus cerebri** of the midbrain.

Having passed through the ventral portion of the pons, corticospinal fibres reach the medulla oblongata, where they form two prominent columns on the ventral surface. These are called the **pyramids** and for this reason the term **pyramidal tract** is used as an alternative name for the corticospinal tract. In the caudal medulla, the fibres of the pyramids undergo subtotal decussation. About 75–90% of fibres decussate and enter the contralateral **lateral corticospinal tract**, which is located in the lateral part of the spinal white matter, deep to the dorsal spinocerebellar tract; 10–25% of pyramidal fibres remain ipsilateral and enter the **ventral corticospinal tract** located lateral to the ventral median fissure. They also decussate near to their termination; as a result, the fibres of the pyramidal tract effectively innervate the contralateral side of the spinal cord.

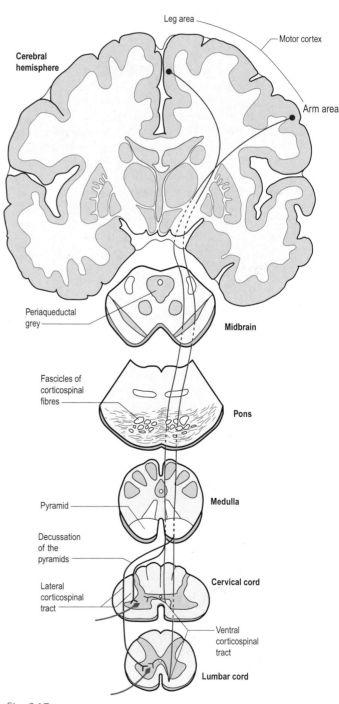

Fig. 8.17 **Corticospinal tracts.**

Approximately 55% of corticospinal neurones terminate at cervical levels, 20% at thoracic and 25% at lumbosacral levels. Fibres terminate extensively in the spinal grey matter. Many of those fibres that originate from the motor cortex terminate in the ventral horn, some making monosynaptic contact with motor neurones.

Rubrospinal tract

The rubrospinal tract originates from the **red nucleus** of the midbrain tegmentum (Fig. 8.18). It exerts control over the tone of limb flexor muscles, being excitatory to the motor neurones of these muscles. Axons leaving the cells of the red nucleus course ventromedially and cross in the **ventral tegmental decussation**, after which they descend to the spinal cord where they lie ventrolateral to, and partly intermingled with, the lateral corticospinal tract.

The red nucleus receives afferent fibres from the motor cortex and from the cerebellum. The rubrospinal tract, therefore, represents a non-pyramidal route by which the motor cortex and cerebellum can influence spinal motor activity.

Tectospinal tract

Tectospinal fibres arise from the **superior colliculus** of the midbrain (Fig. 8.19). Axons pass ventromedially around the periaqueductal grey matter and cross in the **dorsal tegmental decussation**. In the spinal cord, descending tectospinal fibres lie near the ventral median fissure and terminate predominantly in cervical segments. The superior colliculus receives visual input and the tectospinal tract is thought to mediate reflex movements in response to visual stimuli.

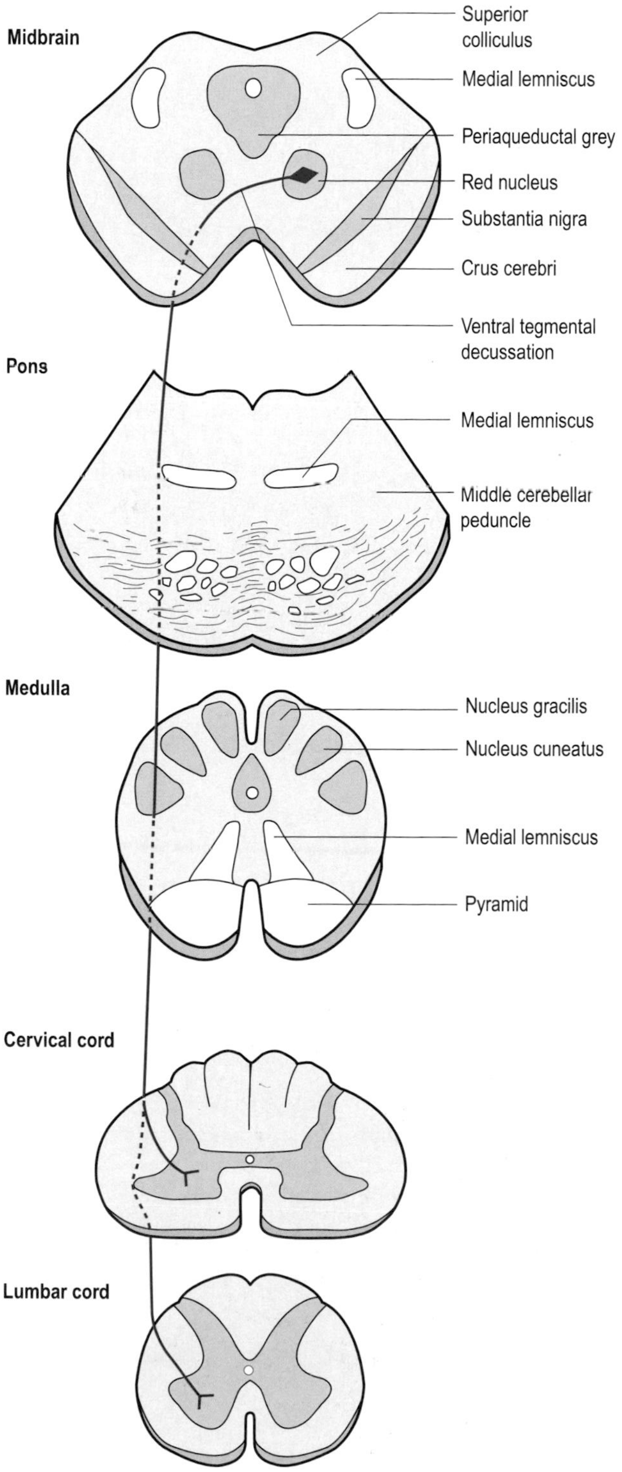

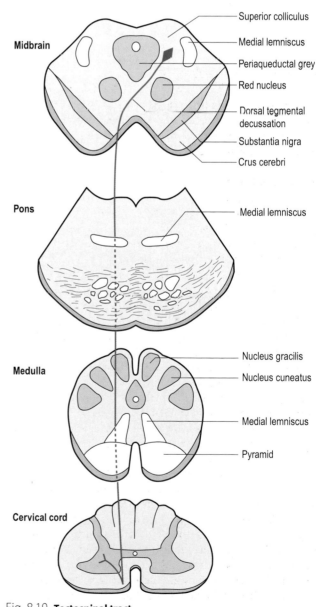

Fig. 8.18 **Rubrospinal tract.**

Fig. 8.19 **Tectospinal tract.**

Vestibulospinal tracts

Vestibulospinal fibres arise from the **vestibular nuclei** situated in the pons and medulla, in and near the floor of the fourth ventricle (Fig. 8.20). The vestibular nuclei receive input from the labyrinthine system by way of the vestibular nerve and from the cerebellum.

Axons from cells of the **lateral vestibular nucleus** (**Deiters' nucleus**) descend ipsilaterally as the **lateral vestibulospinal tract**, which is located in the ventral funiculus. Lateral vestibulospinal tract fibres mediate excitatory influences upon extensor motor neurones. They serve to control extensor muscle tone in the anti-gravity maintenance of posture.

The **medial vestibular nucleus** contributes descending fibres to the ipsilateral **medial longitudinal fasciculus**, also known as the **medial vestibulospinal tract**, which is located adjacent to the ventral median fissure.

Reticulospinal tracts

The reticular formation of the pons and medulla gives rise to reticulospinal fibres. Axons arising from the pontine reticular formation descend ipsilaterally as the **medial (or pontine) reticulospinal tract**. Axons from the medulla descend bilaterally in the **lateral (or medullary) reticulospinal tracts**. Both tracts are located in the ventral funiculus.

Reticulospinal fibres influence voluntary movement, reflex activity and muscle tone by controlling the activity of both alpha and gamma motor neurones. They also mediate pressor and depressor effects upon the circulatory system and are involved in the control of breathing.

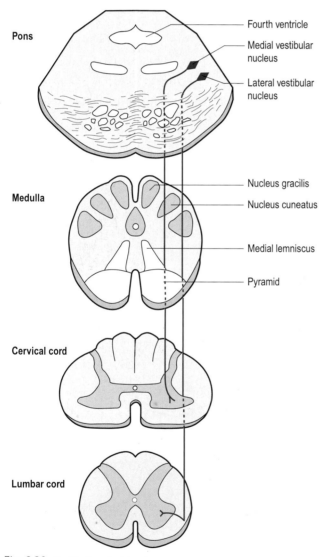

Pons

Medulla

Cervical cord

Lumbar cord

Fourth ventricle

Medial vestibular nucleus

Lateral vestibular nucleus

Nucleus gracilis

Nucleus cuneatus

Medial lemniscus

Pyramid

Fig. 8.20 **Vestibulospinal tracts.**

White matter of the spinal cord: principal descending tracts

- Corticospinal tract controls discrete, skilled movements, particularly of the distal extremities. It originates from motor and sensory cortices. Fibres descend through the internal capsule, crus cerebri and ventral pons to reach the medullary pyramid. Most fibres (75–90%) decussate to form the lateral corticospinal tract, the remainder forming the ventral corticospinal tract.
- Rubrospinal tract controls limb flexor muscles and originates from the red nucleus of the midbrain. Fibres cross in the ventral tegmental decussation.
- Tectospinal tract is involved in reflex responses to visual input. It originates from the contralateral superior colliculus and fibres cross in the dorsal tegmental decussation.
- Vestibulospinal tracts descend from the vestibular nuclei. The lateral tract originates from the ipsilateral lateral vestibular nucleus and mediates excitation of limb extensor muscles.
- Reticulospinal tracts descend from the pons and medulla. They are involved in the control of reflex activities, muscle tone and vital functions.

 ### Lesions of the spinal cord

Focal lesions of the spinal cord and the nerve roots produce clinical manifestations in two ways:

- the lesion destroys function at the segmental level
- the lesion interrupts descending motor and ascending sensory tracts.

Damage to different parts of the spinal cord, therefore, is accompanied by distinctive clinical syndromes, which can be diagrammatically represented (Fig. 8.21 A–E).

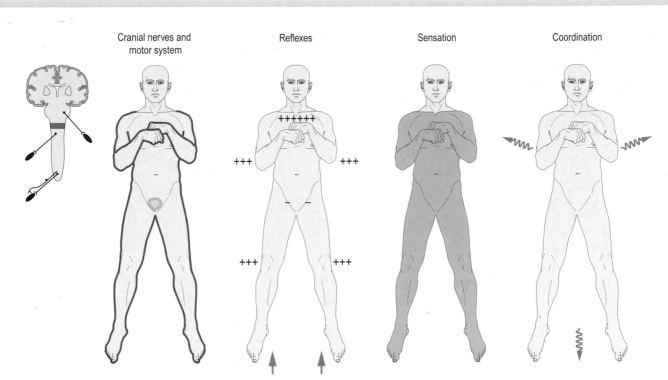

Fig. 8.21A **Upper cervical cord lesion.** A high cervical cord lesion causes spastic tetraplegia with hyperreflexia, extensor plantar responses (upper motor neurone lesion), incontinence, sensory loss below the level of the lesion and 'sensory' ataxia. For key refer to Fig. 1.43.

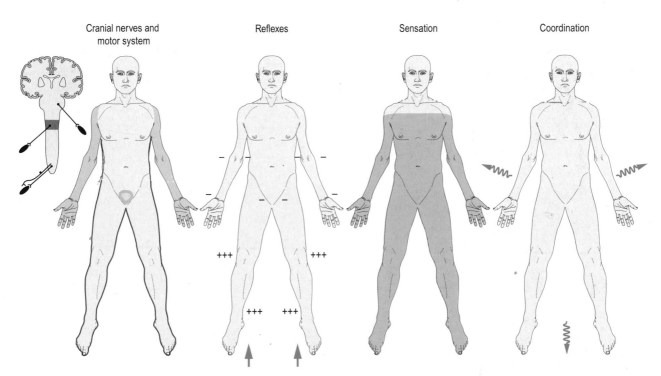

Fig. 8.21B **Lower cervical cord lesion.** A lower cervical cord lesion causes weakness, wasting and fasciculation of muscles, and areflexia of the upper limbs (lower motor neurone lesion). In addition, there is spastic paraparesis, hyperreflexia and extensor plantar responses (upper motor neurone lesion) in the lower limbs, incontinence, sensory loss below the level of the lesion and 'sensory' ataxia. For key refer to Fig. 1.43.

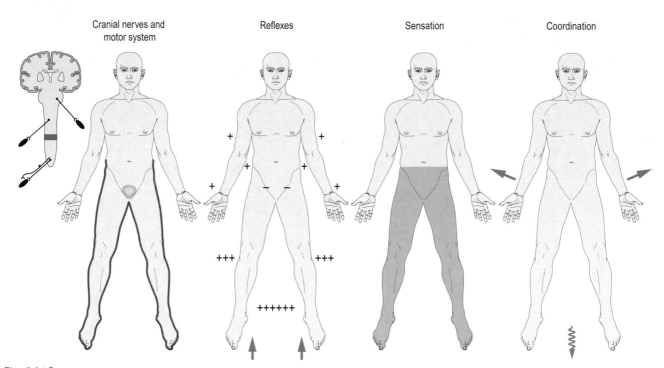

Fig. 8.21C **Thoracic cord lesion.** A thoracic cord lesion causes a spastic paraparesis, hyperreflexia and extensor plantar responses (upper motor neurone lesion), incontinence, sensory loss below the level of the lesion and 'sensory' ataxia. For key refer to Fig. 1.43.

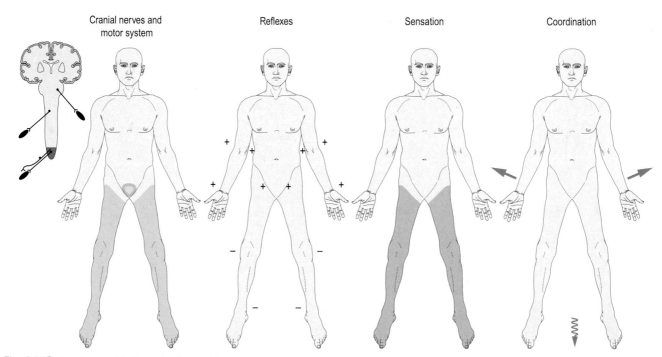

Fig. 8.21D **Lumbar cord lesion.** A lumbar cord lesion causes weakness, wasting and fasciculation of muscles, areflexia of the lower limbs (lower motor neurone lesion), incontinence, sensory loss below the level of the lesion and 'sensory' ataxia. For key refer to Fig. 1.43.

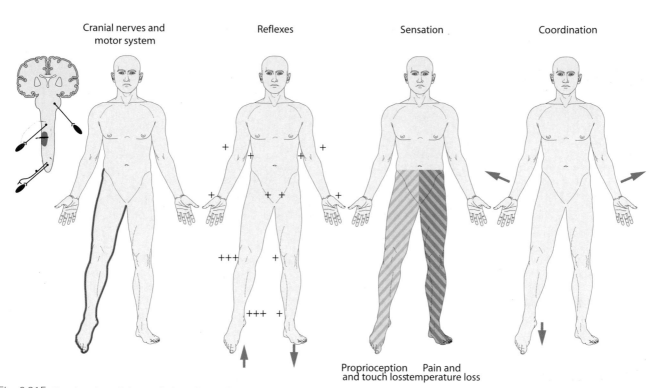

Cranial nerves and motor system Reflexes Sensation Coordination

Proprioception and touch loss   Pain and temperature loss

Fig. 8.21E **Hemisection of the cord gives rise to the Brown-Séquard syndrome.** This is characterised by ipsilateral loss of proprioception and upper motor neurone signs (hemiplegia/monoplegia) plus contralateral loss of pain and temperature sensation. For key refer to Fig. 1.43.

Chapter 9
Brain stem

The brain stem consists of the medulla oblongata, pons and midbrain. The archaic term 'bulb' is applied to the brain stem in compound anatomical names given to nerve fibres originating from, or terminating in, the brain stem (e.g. 'corticobulbar' refers to axons that arise in the cerebral cortex and terminate in the brain stem). It is also used clinically to denote the medulla in such terms as 'bulbar palsy' and 'pseudobulbar palsy', which describe syndromes associated with medullary dysfunction.

The brain stem lies upon the basal portion of the occipital bone (clivus) and is connected to, and largely covered by, the cerebellum. Caudally, the medulla is continuous with the spinal cord at the level of the foramen magnum. Rostrally, the midbrain is continuous with the diencephalon of the forebrain.

The brain stem contains numerous ascending and descending fibre tracts. Some of these pass throughout its whole length, having their origin in the spinal cord or cerebral hemisphere, respectively; others have their origin or termination within brain stem nuclei. Certain of these brain stem nuclei receive fibres from, or send fibres into, cranial nerves, ten pairs of which (III–XII) attach to the surface of the brain stem. These are known as the **cranial nerve nuclei**. In addition, the brain stem contains a complex and heterogeneous matrix of neurones known as the **reticular formation**, within which a number of individually identified nuclei exist. The reticular formation has several important functions, including control over the level of consciousness, the perception of pain and regulation of the cardiovascular and respiratory systems. It also has extensive connections with the cranial nerve nuclei, with the cerebellum, and with brain stem and spinal motor mechanisms, through which it influences movement, posture and muscle tone.

External features of the brain stem

Dorsal surface of the brain stem

The dorsal surface of the brain stem can be viewed if the overlying cerebellum is removed by cutting the three pairs of **peduncles**, or nerve fibre bundles, by which they are attached on each side (Figs 9.1 and 9.2). On the dorsal surface of the medulla, the midline is marked by a dorsal median sulcus, continuous with that of the spinal cord. In the caudal part of the medulla, the **dorsal columns** (**fasciculi gracilis** and **cuneatus**, containing first-order sensory neurones) continue rostrally from the spinal cord to their termination in the **nuclei gracilis** and **cuneatus**, the locations of which are marked by two small elevations, the gracile and cuneate tubercles.

The caudal two-thirds of the medulla contains the rostral continuation of the central canal of the spinal cord and is, therefore, sometimes referred to as the 'closed' portion of the medulla. In passing rostrally, the central canal moves progressively more dorsally until, in the rostral medulla, it opens out into the fourth ventricle. This portion is sometimes referred to as the 'open' medulla. The floor of the fourth ventricle forms a shallow, rhomboid depression on the dorsal surface of the rostral medulla and the pons. The transition from medulla to pons is not clearly delineated on the dorsal surface of the brain stem but, approximately, the caudal third of the floor of the fourth ventricle constitutes the dorsal aspect of the rostral medulla, while the rostral two-thirds of the ventricular floor is made up of the dorsal aspect of the pons. The fourth ventricle is widest at the level of the pontomedullary junction where a **lateral recess** extends to the lateral margin of the brain stem. At this point the small **lateral aperture** (**foramen of Luschka**) provides passage for CSF within the fourth ventricle to reach the subarachnoid space surrounding the brain. The lateral walls of the rostral part of the fourth ventricle are made up of the **superior** and **inferior cerebellar peduncles**, connecting the brain stem with the cerebellum. In the rostral pons, the walls converge until, at the pontomesencephalic junction, the fourth ventricle becomes continuous with a small channel, the **cerebral aqueduct**, which passes throughout the length of the midbrain.

The dorsal aspect of the midbrain is marked by four paired elevations, the **superior** and **inferior colliculi**, which are parts of the visual and auditory systems, respectively. The **trochlear nerve** (IV cranial nerve) emerges immediately caudal to the inferior colliculus.

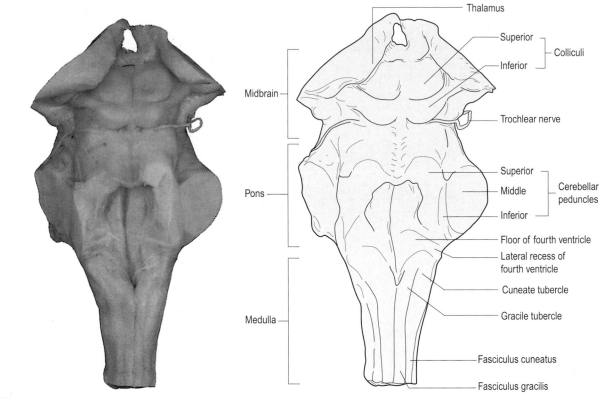

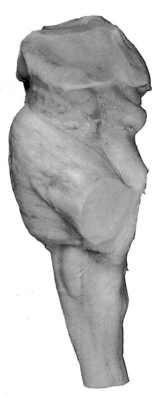

Fig. 9.1 **The dorsal aspect of the brain stem.**

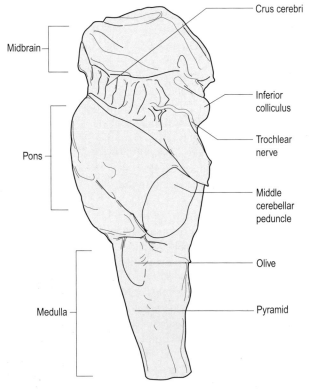

Fig. 9.2 **The lateral aspect of the brain stem.**

Ventral surface of the brain stem

On the ventral surface of the medulla, prominent longitudinal columns, the **pyramids**, run on either side of the ventral median fissure (Figs 9.3 and 9.4). The pyramid gives its name to the underlying **pyramidal** or **corticospinal tract**, which consists of descending fibres originating from the ipsilateral cerebral cortex. In the caudal medulla, 75–90% of these fibres cross over in the **decussation of the pyramids** (Figs 9.3, 9.4 and 9.5), partly obscuring the ventral median fissure as they do so, to form the lateral corticospinal tract of the spinal cord. Lateral to the pyramid lies an elongated elevation, the olive, within which

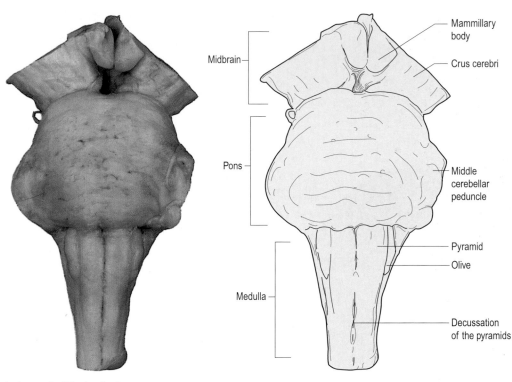

Fig. 9.3 **The ventral aspect of the brain stem.**

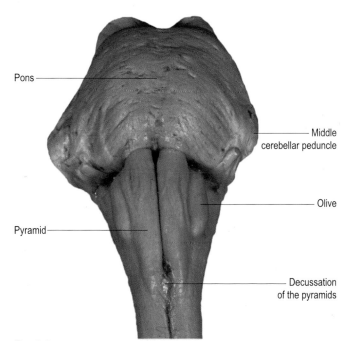

Fig. 9.4 **The ventral aspect of the brain stem showing the decussation of the pyramids.**

lies the **inferior olivary nucleus**. This has connections primarily with the cerebellum and is involved in the control of movement.

The transition from medulla to pons is clearly delineated on the ventral surface of the brain stem. The ventral part of the pons is dominated by a transverse system of fibres (the **transverse pontine fibres** or **pontocerebellar fibres**) that originate from cells in the ventral pons (**pontine nuclei**) and pass through the contralateral **middle cerebellar peduncle** to enter the cerebellar hemisphere. The pontine

nuclei receive corticopontine fibres from the cerebral cortex (including the motor cortex) and constitute an important connection between cerebral and cerebellar cortices involved in the coordination of movement. The massive system of transverse pontine fibres obscures the underlying corticospinal tract.

The ventral surface of the midbrain consists, on either side, of a huge column of descending fibres, the **crus cerebri** or **basis pedunculi**. In the midline, the two crura cerebri are separated by a depression called the interpeduncular fossa. The crus cerebri is continuous rostrally with the internal capsule of the cerebral hemisphere (Fig. 1.25) and consists of corticobulbar and corticospinal fibres that have left the cerebral hemisphere via the internal capsule on their way to the brain stem and spinal cord. They are primarily motor in function.

External features of the brain stem

- ■ The brain stem consists of the medulla oblongata, pons and midbrain.
- ■ On the dorsal aspect of the brain stem can be seen the dorsal columns, the floor of the fourth ventricle and the superior and inferior colliculi.
- ■ The dorsal aspect of the rostral medulla and the pons form the floor of the fourth ventricle; the lateral and median apertures of the fourth ventricle permit the passage of CSF into the subarachnoid space. The cerebral aqueduct runs through the midbrain, beneath the colliculi.
- ■ On the ventral aspect of the brain stem can be seen the pyramids, transverse pontine fibres and the crura cerebri.
- ■ The inferior, middle and superior cerebellar peduncles connect the cerebellum to the medulla, pons and midbrain, respectively.

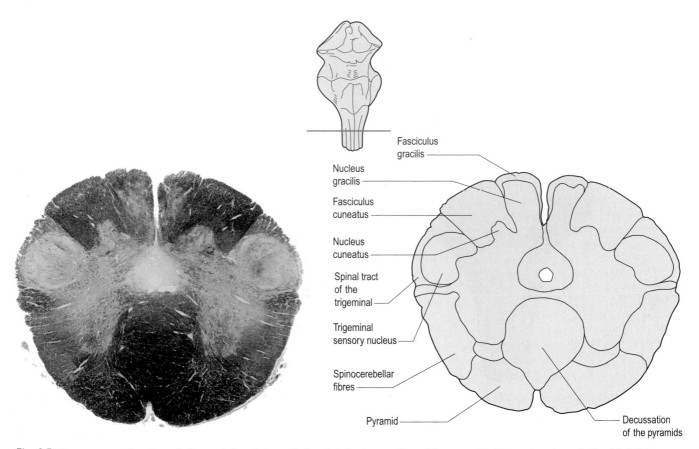

Fig. 9.5 **Transverse section through the caudal medulla at the level of the decussation of the pyramids.** The sections shown in Figs 9.5–9.13 have been stained by the Weigert–Pal method. Areas rich in nerve fibres stain darkly, while areas rich in cell bodies are relatively pale.

Internal structure of the brain stem

Caudal medulla

At the transition from spinal cord to medulla, the pattern of grey and white matter undergoes considerable rearrangement (Fig. 9.5). The ventral horn becomes much attenuated. The dorsal horn is replaced by the caudal part of the **trigeminal sensory nucleus (nucleus of the spinal tract of the trigeminal nerve)**. The trigeminal sensory nucleus is regarded as the brain stem homologue of the dorsal horn since it receives primary afferent fibres conveying general sensation from the head, which enter the brain stem in the trigeminal nerve. It is a large nucleus that extends the whole length of the brain stem and into the upper segments of the spinal cord. This latter, caudal part of the trigeminal nucleus is particularly associated with the modalities of pain and temperature. The trigeminal nerve attaches to the pons and, therefore, fibres that terminate in the parts of the trigeminal nucleus caudal to this level descend in a tract (**the spinal tract of the trigeminal**) which lies immediately superficial to the nucleus.

In the ventral medulla, the majority of fibres of the pyramid undergo decussation and then pass laterally, dorsally and caudally to form the lateral corticospinal tract.

Mid-medulla

On the ventral surface of the mid-medulla the pyramids are prominent, above their decussation. On the dorsal surface, the dorsal columns reach their termination in the gracile and cuneate nuclei which appear beneath their respective tracts (Fig. 9.6). The dorsal columns consist of first-order sensory

neurones; the cell bodies of these neurones lie in the dorsal root ganglia of spinal nerves and have central processes that ascended ipsilaterally through the cord and into the medulla. They terminate in the nucleus gracilis and cuneatus upon the cell bodies of second-order neurones. The axons of the latter course ventrally and medially as **internal arcuate fibres**, decussating in the midline. Thereafter, they turn rostrally forming a distinct tract, the **medial lemniscus**, that runs through the rostral medulla, the pons and midbrain to terminate in the ventral posterior nucleus of the thalamus.

Rostral medulla

On the ventral surface of the medulla, the pyramids remain conspicuous. Immediately dorsal to the medial aspect of the pyramid lies the medial lemniscus, on either side of the midline (Fig. 9.7). Dorsolateral to the pyramid and lateral to the medial lemniscus is the **inferior olivary nucleus**, lying within the prominence of the olive. The inferior olivary nucleus has roughly the form of a crenated bag with an opening, or hilum, facing medially, through which afferent and efferent fibres pass. The nucleus is concerned with the control of movement and receives afferents from the motor and sensory cortices of the cerebral hemisphere and from the red nucleus of the midbrain. Its main efferent connection is to the cerebellum via the inferior cerebellar peduncle. Within the cerebellum, axons originating from the inferior olivary nucleus, known as climbing fibres, end in excitatory synapses in the dentate nucleus and upon Purkinje cells of the cerebellar cortex.

Dorsal to the inferior olivary nucleus and lateral to the medial lemniscus lie second-order sensory fibres ascending

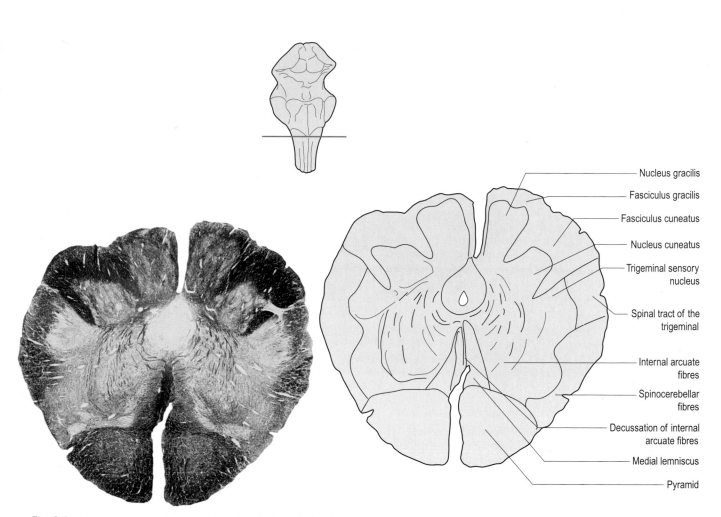

Fig. 9.6 **Transverse section through the mid-medulla at the level of the sensory decussation.**

Labels (top to bottom, right side):
- Nucleus gracilis
- Fasciculus gracilis
- Fasciculus cuneatus
- Nucleus cuneatus
- Trigeminal sensory nucleus
- Spinal tract of the trigeminal
- Internal arcuate fibres
- Spinocerebellar fibres
- Decussation of internal arcuate fibres
- Medial lemniscus
- Pyramid

to the ventral posterior thalamus from the trigeminal nucleus (the **trigeminothalamic tract**) and from the spinal cord (spinothalamic fibres, referred to in the brain stem as the **spinal lemniscus**).

The dorsal surface of the rostral medulla forms part of the floor of the fourth ventricle. Both immediately and deep beneath the floor of the ventricle lie a number of cranial nerve nuclei, some of which can be clearly identified in simply stained sections, others of which cannot. Immediately beneath the ventricular floor, just lateral to the midline, lies the **hypoglossal nucleus**, which contains motor neurones innervating the muscles of the tongue via the hypoglossal nerve. Lateral to the hypoglossal nucleus lies the **dorsal (motor) nucleus of the vagus**, containing preganglionic parasympathetic neurones that run in the vagus nerve. The most caudal aspect of the ventricular floor is known as the **area postrema**. At this point the blood–brain barrier, which limits the passage of certain chemicals from the blood to the brain, is absent. This region is the central site of action of substances that cause vomiting (emetics). In the lateral part of the floor of the fourth ventricle are located the **vestibular nuclei**, which receive primary afferent fibres from the vestibular nerve. Ventromedial to the hypoglossal nucleus, close to the midline, is located the **medial longitudinal fasciculus**. This consists of both ascending and descending fibres and can be identified also in the pons and midbrain. Within the brain stem, it links the vestibular nuclei with the nuclei supplying the extraocular muscles (abducens,

trochlear and oculomotor nuclei) and subserves the coordination of head and eye movements.

The dorsolateral part of the rostral medulla is dominated by the inferior cerebellar peduncle, or **restiform body**. This consists of fibres passing between the medulla and the cerebellum. Prominent amongst these are olivocerebellar fibres, connections between the vestibular nuclei and the cerebellum, and the fibres of the dorsal spinocerebellar tract, conveying proprioceptive information from the limbs. On the dorsal and lateral aspects of the inferior cerebellar peduncle lie the dorsal and ventral **cochlear nuclei**, which receive afferent fibres from the cochlear nerve. Deep beneath the ventricular floor, just dorsal to the inferior olivary nucleus, is located the **nucleus ambiguus**. This sends motor fibres into the glossopharyngeal, vagus and accessory nerves and, thence, to the muscles of the pharynx and larynx.

Pons

The pons may be divided into a ventral, or basal, portion and a dorsal portion, also known as the **tegmentum**. The ventral portion is marked by numerous transversely oriented fascicles of pontocerebellar fibres that originate from scattered cell groups, the **pontine nuclei**, and pass to the contralateral side of the cerebellum through the massive middle cerebellar peduncle (**brachium pontis**) (Figs 9.8–9.10). Corticospinal fibres (which continue into the medullary pyramid) appear as small, separate bundles running longitudinally between the fascicles of transverse pontine fibres.

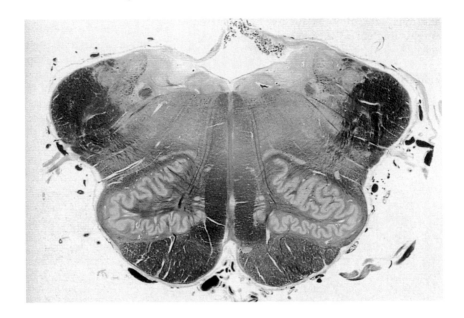

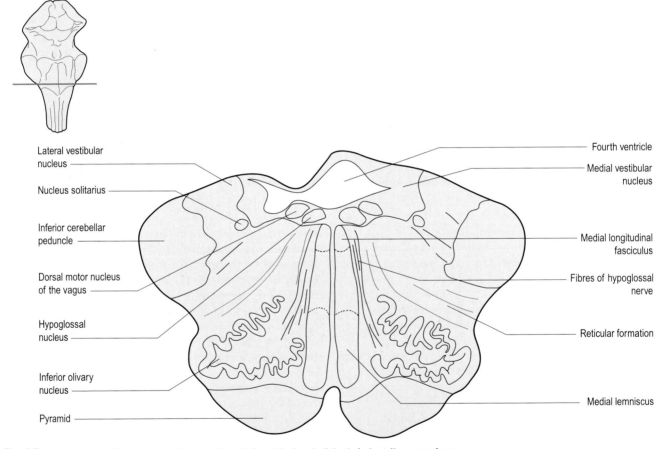

Lateral vestibular nucleus

Nucleus solitarius

Inferior cerebellar peduncle

Dorsal motor nucleus of the vagus

Hypoglossal nucleus

Inferior olivary nucleus

Pyramid

Fourth ventricle

Medial vestibular nucleus

Medial longitudinal fasciculus

Fibres of hypoglossal nerve

Reticular formation

Medial lemniscus

Fig. 9.7 **Transverse section through the rostral medulla at the level of the inferior olivary nucleus.**

The ascending fibres of the medial lemniscus become separated from the pyramid and displaced dorsally, together with the spinal lemniscus and trigeminothalamic tract, by intervening transverse pontocerebellar fibres. The medial lemniscus also rotates through 90° so that it lies almost horizontally, marking the boundary between ventral and tegmental portions of the pons. In the caudal pons (Fig. 9.8), an additional group of transversely running fibres is located ventral to the ascending lemniscal fibres but dorsal to the pontocerebellar fibres. This is the **trapezoid body**, which consists of acoustic fibres crossing the brain stem from the cochlear nuclei. They ascend into the midbrain as the **lateral lemniscus** and terminate in the inferior colliculus.

Beneath the floor of the fourth ventricle, in the pontine tegmentum, lie a number of cranial nerve nuclei. These include the **abducens nucleus** (lateral rectus muscle), the **facial motor nucleus** (muscles of facial expression) and the **trigeminal motor nucleus** (muscles of mastication), which each supply motor axons to their respective cranial nerves. Also the trigeminal sensory nucleus, already

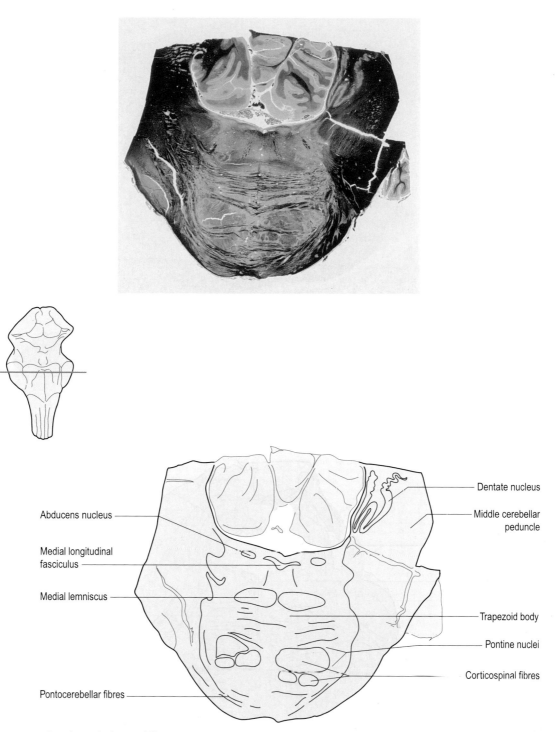

Fig. 9.8 **Transverse section through the caudal pons.**

encountered in the medulla, reaches its maximum extent in the pons, adjacent to the origin of the trigeminal nerve.

In the rostral part of the pons (Fig. 9.10) the superior cerebellar peduncles form the lateral walls of the fourth ventricle, the thin superior medullary velum spanning between them to form its roof. The superior peduncle contains some cerebellar afferent fibres, such as the ventral spinocerebellar tract, which conveys proprioceptive information from the limbs. It consists mainly, however, of ascending cerebellar efferents concerned with the coordination of movement that are destined for the red nucleus of the midbrain and the ventral lateral nucleus of the thalamus. The superior cerebellar peduncles converge towards the midline as they pass into the midbrain.

Midbrain

The midbrain is formally divided into dorsal and ventral portions at the level of the cerebral aqueduct. The dorsal portion is known as the **tectum**, which consists largely of the **inferior** and **superior colliculi** (**corpora quadrigemina**). The ventral portion of the midbrain is known as the **tegmentum**. It is bounded ventrally by the massive fibre system of the crus cerebri. The term **cerebral peduncle** is sometimes used as a synonym for crus cerebri, but strictly speaking, the cerebral peduncle refers to the whole midbrain, on either side, excluding the tectum.

In the caudal part of the midbrain, the inferior colliculus constitutes part of the **ascending acoustic** (**auditory**) **projection**. Ascending auditory fibres run in the lateral

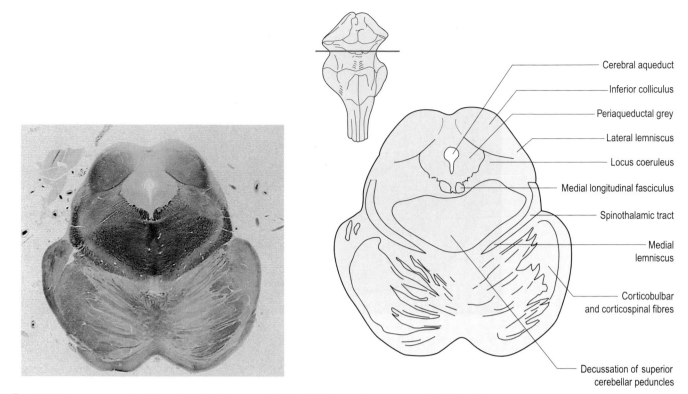

Fig. 9.11 **Transverse section through the brain stem at the level of the pontine–mesencephalic junction.**

Labels (Fig. 9.11):
- Cerebral aqueduct
- Inferior colliculus
- Periaqueductal grey
- Lateral lemniscus
- Locus coeruleus
- Medial longitudinal fasciculus
- Spinothalamic tract
- Medial lemniscus
- Corticobulbar and corticospinal fibres
- Decussation of superior cerebellar peduncles

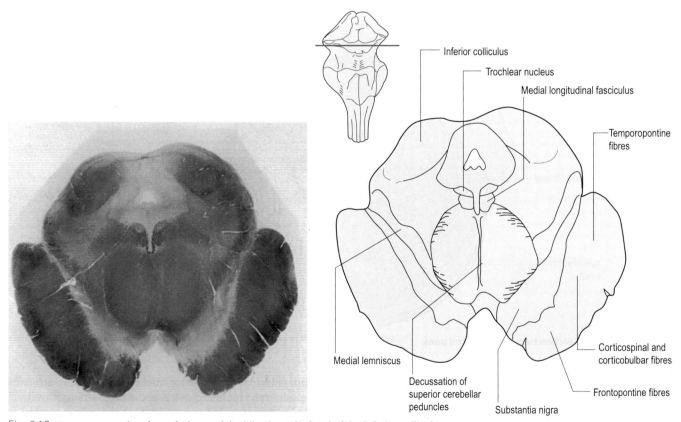

Fig. 9.12 **Transverse section through the caudal midbrain at the level of the inferior colliculus.**

Labels (Fig. 9.12):
- Inferior colliculus
- Trochlear nucleus
- Medial longitudinal fasciculus
- Temporopontine fibres
- Corticospinal and corticobulbar fibres
- Frontopontine fibres
- Substantia nigra
- Decussation of superior cerebellar peduncles
- Medial lemniscus

The most ventral part of the midbrain tegmentum is occupied by the **substantia nigra**. A subdivision of this nucleus, known as the **pars compacta**, consists of pigmented, melanin-containing neurones that synthesise dopamine as their transmitter. These neurones project to the caudate nucleus and putamen of the basal ganglia in the forebrain. Degeneration of the pars compacta of the substantia nigra is associated with Parkinson's disease. The other, non-pigmented, subdivision of the substantia nigra is called the **pars reticulata**. It is considered to be a functional homologue of the medial segment of the globus pallidus, which is also part of the basal ganglia (Chapter 14).

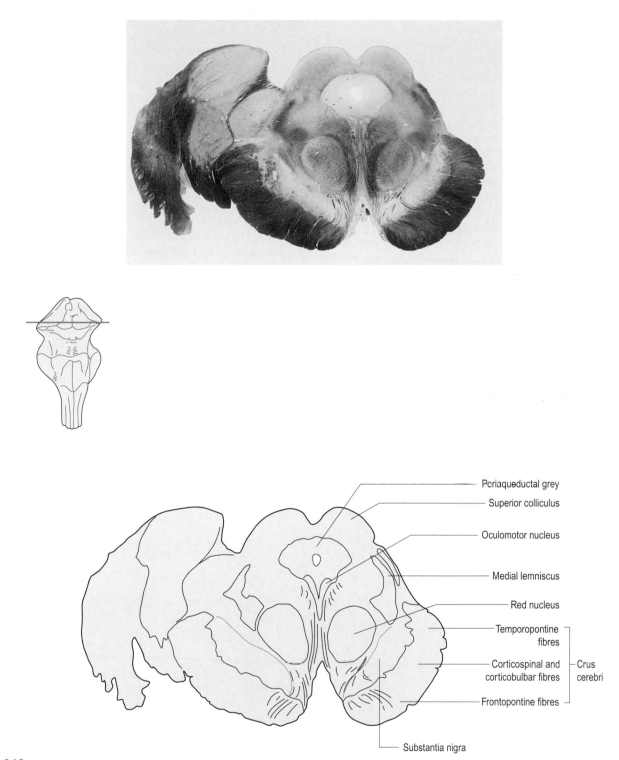

Fig. 9.13 **Transverse section through the rostral midbrain at the level of the superior colliculus.**

Periaqueductal grey
Superior colliculus
Oculomotor nucleus
Medial lemniscus
Red nucleus
Temporopontine fibres ⎤
Corticospinal and corticobulbar fibres ⎬ Crus cerebri
Frontopontine fibres ⎦
Substantia nigra

Ventral to the substantia nigra lies the massive crus cerebri. This consists entirely of descending cortical efferent fibres that have left the cerebral hemisphere by traversing the internal capsule. Approximately the middle 50% of the crus consists of **corticobulbar** and **corticospinal fibres**. The corticobulbar fibres end predominantly in or near the motor cranial nerve nuclei of the brain stem. The corticospinal (pyramidal) fibres traverse the pons to enter the medullary pyramid and, thence, the corticospinal tract.

On either side of the corticobulbar and corticospinal fibres, the crus cerebri contains corticopontine fibres that originate from widespread regions of the cerebral cortex and terminate in the pontine nuclei of the ventral pons. From the pontine nuclei connections are established with the cerebellum, via the middle cerebellar peduncle, which are involved in the coordination of movement.

Reticular formation

The reticular formation consists of a complex matrix of neurones that extends throughout the length of the brain stem. This is, in phylogenetic terms, a relatively old part of the brain stem and its neurones fulfil a number of important functions, some of which are necessary for survival. The reticular formation has widespread afferent and efferent

Brain stem lesions

A unilateral brain stem lesion caused by stroke, tumour or multiple sclerosis causes ipsilateral cranial nerve dysfunction, contralateral spastic hemiparesis, hyperreflexia and an extensor plantar response (upper motor neurone lesion), contralateral hemisensory loss and ipsilateral incoordination (Fig. 9.14). A bilateral lesion destroys the 'vital centres' for respiration and the circulation, leading to coma and death. Multiple sclerosis can affect eye movements through demyelination of the medial longitudinal fasciculus, which interferes with conjugate ocular deviation. Typically, on horizontal gaze, the abducting eye moves normally but the adducting eye fails to follow. Adduction is preserved on convergence. **Internuclear ophthalmoplegia** is the term used to describe this disorder (Fig. 9.15).

Internal structure of the brain stem

■ Cranial nerves III–XII attach to the brain stem, their fibres either originating from, or terminating in, the cranial nerve nuclei.
■ The reticular formation controls the level of consciousness, the cardiovascular system and the respiratory system.
■ Ascending sensory systems pass through the brain stem en route to the thalamus. First-order proprioceptive fibres in the dorsal columns relay in the dorsal column nuclei. Second-order fibres decussate to form the medial lemniscus. Spinothalamic fibres form the spinal lemniscus.
■ Descending fibre systems both pass through the brain stem and originate within it.
■ The corticospinal tract runs through the crus cerebri, the basal part of the pons and the medullary pyramid; 75–90% of fibres cross in the pyramidal decussation to form the lateral corticospinal tract.
■ The reticular formation, red nucleus and vestibular nuclei give rise to descending fibres that pass to the spinal cord.

connections with other parts of the CNS, which reflect its complex and multimodal functions. Some reticular neurones have long axons that ascend and descend for considerable distances within the brain stem, allowing profuse interaction with other neuronal systems. Within the reticular formation a number of individual nuclei are recognised. Some functions are subserved, however, by more dispersed networks that do not correspond exactly to anatomically

identified nuclei. The latter applies to the so-called respiratory and cardiovascular centres. These consist of diffuse neuronal networks located within the medullary and caudal pontine reticular formation that control respiratory movements and cardiovascular function.

Descending **reticulospinal tracts** originate from the medullary and pontine reticular formation (Chapter 8).

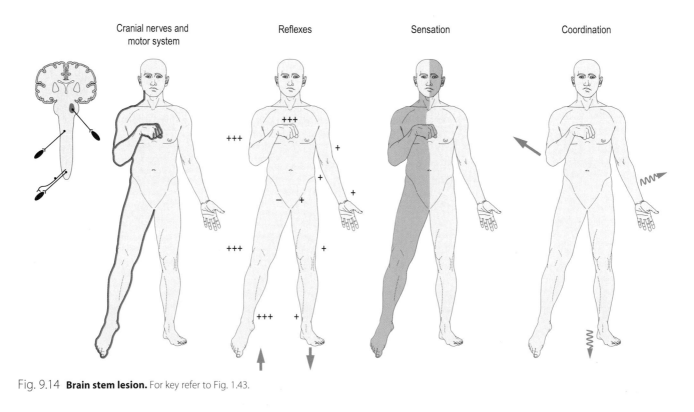

Fig. 9.14 **Brain stem lesion.** For key refer to Fig. 1.43.

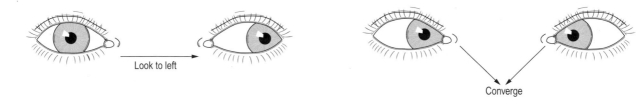

Fig. 9.15 **Internuclear ophthalmoplegia.**

These predominantly influence muscle tone and posture. Some of the ascending fibres of the reticular formation constitute the **reticular activating system**. These neurones receive input, either directly or indirectly, from multiple sensory sources. Through the intermediary of thalamic nuclei, they cause activation of the cerebral cortex and heightened arousal.

The **raphe nuclei** are a group of midline nuclei that extend throughout the length of the brain stem. Many of the neurones of these nuclei are serotonergic, utilising serotonin (5-hydroxytryptamine, 5-HT) as their transmitter. Their axons are widely distributed throughout the CNS. In particular, ascending fibres to forebrain structures are involved in the neural mechanisms of sleep, and descending fibres to the spinal cord are involved in the modulation of nociceptive mechanisms.

The **locus coeruleus** is a group of pigmented neurones that lies in the brain stem tegmentum of the caudal midbrain and rostral pons. It is the principal noradrenergic cell group of the brain. It projects to many areas of the CNS. Ascending fibres project to the cerebellum, hypothalamus, thalamus, limbic structures and cerebral cortex. Descending fibres project widely throughout the brain stem and spinal cord. The locus coeruleus, like the raphe nuclei, has been implicated in the neural mechanisms regulating sleep, particularly REM (rapid eye movement) sleep.

Chapter 10
Cranial nerves and cranial nerve nuclei

There are twelve, bilaterally paired, cranial nerves; these carry afferent and efferent fibres between the brain and peripheral structures, principally of the head and neck. The cranial nerves are individually named and numbered (Roman numerals) according to the rostrocaudal sequence in which they attach to the brain (Fig. 10.1):

I olfactory	III oculomotor
II optic	IV trochlear
V trigeminal	IX glossopharyngeal
VI abducens	X vagus
VII facial	XI accessory
VIII vestibulocochlear	XII hypoglossal

The first two cranial nerves attach directly to the forebrain, while the rest attach to the brain stem. The olfactory system is closely associated, both structurally and functionally, with parts of the forebrain collectively referred to as the limbic system; these, including cranial nerve I, are considered together in Chapter 16. The visual system and cranial nerve II are described in Chapter 15. Cranial nerves III–XII are associated with various nuclei within the brain stem, called the cranial nerve nuclei, which either receive cranial nerve afferents or contain the cell bodies of efferent neurones that have axons leaving the brain in cranial nerves. The locations of these nuclei are illustrated in Figure 10.2.

Cranial nerve nuclei

Afferent nuclei

Fibres carrying general sensory information (touch, pressure, pain, temperature) from the head enter the brain through the trigeminal nerve at the level of the pons and terminate in

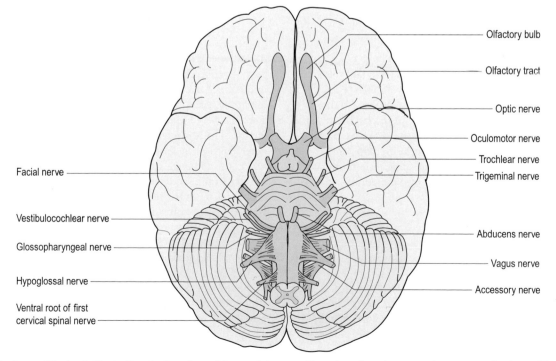

Fig. 10.1 **The base of the brain illustrating the locations of the cranial nerves.** The points of attachment are shown, except for the trochlear nerve, which arises from the dorsal aspect of the brain stem.

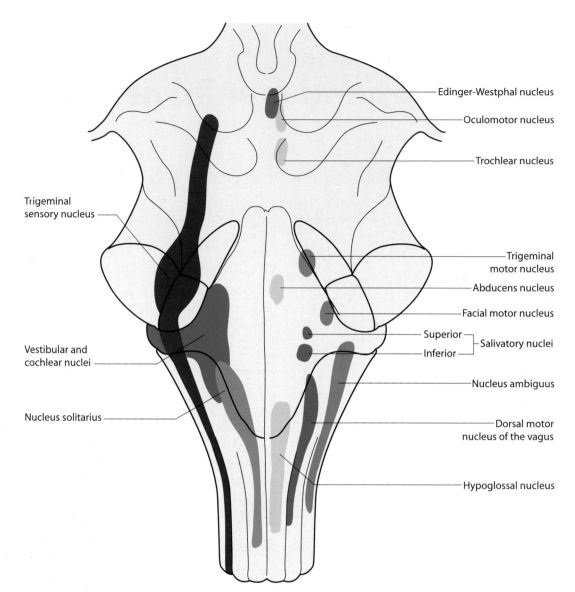

Fig. 10.2 **The brain stem viewed from the dorsal aspect.** The diagram illustrates the locations of the afferent cranial nerve nuclei (left) and the efferent cranial nerve nuclei (right). On the right, nuclei shaded in the same colour share a common embryological origin.

the **trigeminal sensory nucleus**. This is a large nucleus that extends the whole length of the brain stem and caudally into the cervical spinal cord. Fibres conveying the special senses of hearing and motion/positional sense run in the vestibulocochlear nerve. They terminate in the **cochlear** and **vestibular nuclei**, respectively, which are located in the medulla, in and near to the lateral part of the floor of the fourth ventricle. Visceral afferents, including taste fibres, terminate in the **nucleus solitarius** of the medulla.

Efferent nuclei

On the basis of their embryological derivation, the efferent cranial nerve nuclei can be divided into three groups, each lying in a discontinuous longitudinal column.

Nuclei of the somatic efferent cell column

The somatic efferent cell column lies near to the midline and consists of the nuclei of the III, IV, VI and XII nerves. The **oculomotor nucleus** lies in the ventral apex of the periaqueductal grey of the midbrain at the level of the superior colliculus. Its efferent fibres run in the oculomotor nerve to innervate the levator palpebrae superioris and all of

the extraocular muscles, except the superior oblique and lateral rectus. The **trochlear nucleus** also lies in the midbrain, at the ventral border of the periaqueductal grey, but at the level of the inferior colliculus. Fibres leave in the trochlear nerve to innervate the superior oblique muscle of the eye. The **abducens nucleus** is located in the caudal pons beneath the floor of the fourth ventricle. Its efferents run in the abducens nerve and innervate the lateral rectus muscle. In the medulla lies the **hypoglossal nucleus**, which innervates the intrinsic and extrinsic muscles of the tongue via the hypoglossal nerve.

Nuclei of the branchiomotor cell column

The branchiomotor cell column innervates striated muscles derived from the branchial arches. In the tegmentum of the mid-pons is located the **trigeminal motor nucleus**, which supplies fibres to the trigeminal nerve and innervates the muscles of mastication, tensor tympani, tensor veli palitini, mylohyoid and the anterior belly of the digastric muscle. In the caudal pontine tegmentum lies the **facial motor nucleus**. This innervates the muscles of facial expression and the stapedius muscle via the facial nerve. Within the

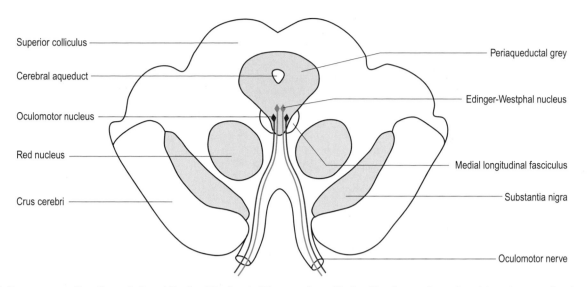

Fig. 10.3 **Transverse section through the midbrain at the level of the superior colliculus.** The diagram shows the origin and course of oculomotor nerve fibres within the brain stem.

medulla lies the **nucleus ambiguus**. This long nucleus sends motor fibres in the glossopharyngeal, vagus and cranial part of the accessory nerve to innervate muscles of the pharynx and larynx.

Nuclei of the parasympathetic cell column

The parasympathetic cell column consists of preganglionic parasympathetic neurones that send axons into the III, VII, IX and X cranial nerves. The most rostral cell group constitutes the **Edinger–Westphal nucleus**, which lies in the midbrain periaqueductal grey matter adjacent to the oculomotor nucleus. Its axons leave in the oculomotor nerve and pass to the ciliary ganglion, from which postganglionic fibres innervate the sphincter pupillae and ciliary muscles within the eye. In the pontine tegmentum lie two cell groups, the **superior** and **inferior salivatory nuclei**. The superior salivatory nucleus supplies preganglionic fibres to the facial nerve that terminate in the pterygopalatine and submandibular ganglia. Postganglionic fibres from the pterygopalatine ganglion innervate the lacrimal gland and the nasal and oral mucous membranes. Those from the submandibular ganglion innervate the submandibular and sublingual salivary glands.

The inferior salivatory nucleus sends preganglionic fibres into the glossopharyngeal nerve. These terminate in the otic ganglion, which in turn sends postganglionic axons to the parotid salivary gland. The largest preganglionic parasympathetic cell group lies in the medulla and constitutes the **dorsal motor nucleus of the vagus**. Its rostral portion lies immediately beneath the floor of the fourth ventricle, lateral to the hypoglossal nucleus. Fibres leave in the vagus nerve and are widely distributed to thoracic and abdominal viscera.

Cranial nerves

III: Oculomotor nerve

The oculomotor nerve carries the majority of somatic motor neurones that innervate extraocular muscles and are responsible for moving the eye. It also contains preganglionic

parasympathetic neurones that, via the intermediary of the ciliary ganglion, control the smooth muscle within the eye.

The motor neurones serving the extraocular muscles have their cell bodies in the **oculomotor nucleus**, which lies at the base of the periaqueductal grey of the midbrain at the level of the superior colliculus (Fig. 10.3). Preganglionic parasympathetic neurones arise from the nearby Edinger–Westphal nucleus. Fibres from both sources course ventrally through the midbrain tegmentum, many of them traversing the red nucleus, to exit on the medial aspect of the crus cerebri, within the interpeduncular fossa (Fig. 10.4). The oculomotor nerve passes between the posterior cerebral and superior cerebellar arteries, then runs anteriorly, lying in the wall of the cavernous sinus, before gaining access to the orbit through the superior orbital fissure. The oculomotor nerve supplies all of the extraocular muscles, with the exception of the superior oblique and lateral rectus and,

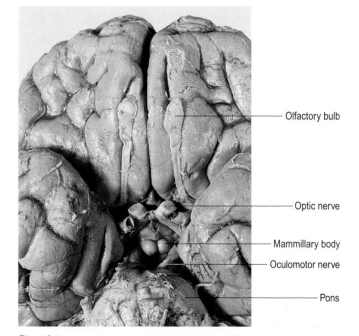

Fig. 10.4 **Ventral aspect of the brain showing the points of attachment of cranial nerves I, II and III.**

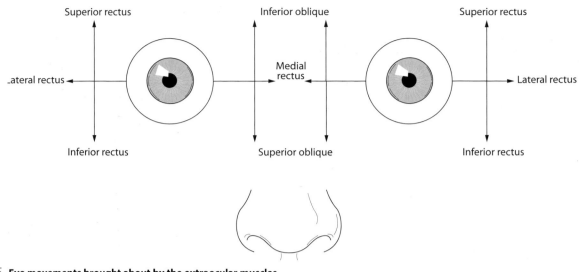

Fig. 10.5 **Eye movements brought about by the extraocular muscles.**

thus, functions to elevate, depress and adduct the eyeball (Fig. 10.5). It also innervates the striated muscle of the levator palpebrae superioris. Preganglionic parasympathetic neurones terminate in the ciliary ganglion. From here postganglionic neurones run in the **short ciliary nerves** to innervate the sphincter (constrictor) pupillae muscle of the iris and the ciliary muscle contained within the ciliary body.

Pupillary light reflex

The amount of light entering the eye is regulated by the size of the pupil. Illumination of the retina causes constriction of the pupil through contraction of the sphincter pupillae muscle of the iris, thus reducing the amount of light reaching the retina. This is known as the **direct light reflex** (Fig. 10.6). Even if only one retina is illuminated (e.g. during clinical examination) the pupils of both eyes constrict. The constriction of the pupil of the non-illuminated eye is called the **consensual light reflex**. The afferent limb of the light reflex consists of a small contingent of optic tract fibres that pass directly from the eye to the **pretectal area**, just rostral to the superior colliculus, rather than the lateral geniculate nucleus of the thalamus (see also Chapter 15). Neurones of

the pretectal area project bilaterally to the Edinger–Westphal nuclei, from which efferent fibres leave in the oculomotor nerve.

Accommodation reflex

Fixation upon a nearby object, by convergence of the optic axes, involves concomitant contraction of the ciliary muscles to increase the convexity of the lens, thus focusing the image. It is also accompanied by pupillary constriction. The phenomenon involves the visual cortex, with corticobulbar fibres activating the parasympathetic neurones of the Edinger–Westphal nuclei bilaterally.

IV: Trochlear nerve

The trochlear nerve contains only somatic motor neurones. These arise in the **trochlear nucleus**, which lies in the midbrain periaqueductal grey at the level of the inferior colliculus (Fig. 10.7). Axons pass dorsally, around the periaqueductal grey, and cross the midline. The trochlear nerve emerges from the dorsal aspect of the brain stem (the only cranial nerve to do so) just caudal to the inferior colliculus (Fig. 10.8). The nerve courses round the cerebral

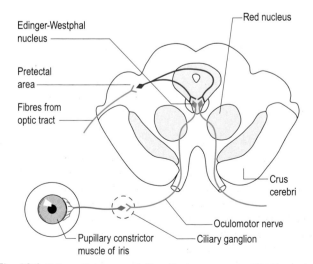

Fig. 10.6 **Schematic representation of a transverse section through the most rostral part of the midbrain.** The diagram shows the pathways involved in the pupillary light reflex.

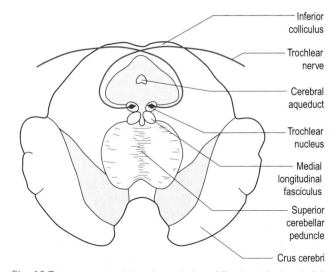

Fig. 10.7 **Transverse section through the midbrain at the level of the inferior colliculus.** The diagram shows the location of the trochlear nucleus and the course of trochlear nerve fibres.

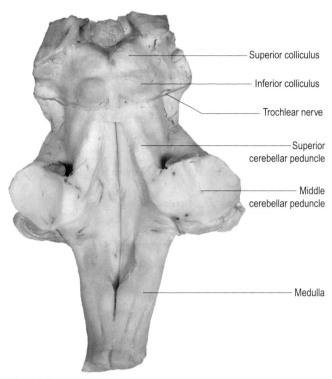

Fig. 10.8 **Dorsal aspect of the brain stem, after removal of the cerebellum, showing the origin of the cranial nerve IV.**

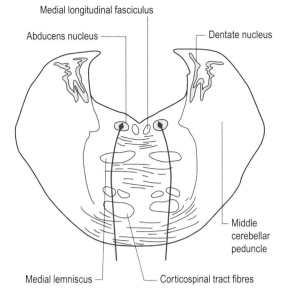

Fig. 10.10 **Transverse section through the caudal pons.** The diagram shows the location of the abducens nucleus and the course of abducens nerve fibres.

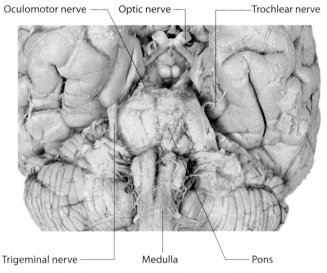

Fig. 10.9 **Ventral aspect of the brain showing cranial nerves III, IV and V.**

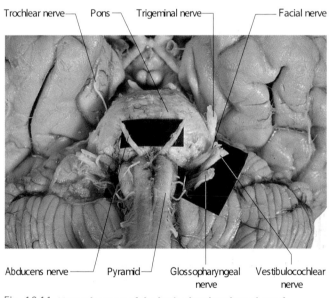

Fig. 10.11 **Ventral aspect of the brain showing the points of attachment of cranial nerves VI to IX.**

peduncle to gain the ventral aspect of the brain (Fig. 10.9), passing between the posterior cerebral and superior cerebellar arteries, as does the oculomotor nerve. It then runs anteriorly, lying in the lateral wall of the cavernous sinus and enters the orbit through the superior orbital fissure. It supplies just one muscle, the **superior oblique**, which moves the eyeball downwards and medially.

VI: Abducens nerve

The abducens, like the trochlear nerve, contains only somatic motor neurones. The cell bodies of origin are located in the **abducens nucleus**, which lies beneath the floor of the fourth ventricle in the caudal pons (Fig. 10.10). Fibres pass ventrally through the pons and emerge from the ventral

surface of the brain stem at the junction between the pons and the pyramid of the medulla (Fig. 10.11). The nerve then passes anteriorly, through the cavernous sinus, enters the orbit through the superior orbital fissure and supplies the lateral rectus muscle, which abducts the eye.

V: Trigeminal nerve

The trigeminal nerve has both sensory and motor components. It is the main sensory nerve for the head and, additionally, innervates the muscles of mastication. It attaches to the brain stem as two adjacent roots (a large sensory and a smaller motor) on the ventrolateral aspect of the pons, where this merges with the middle cerebellar peduncle (Figs 10.1, 10.9 and 10.11).

The sensory fibres of the trigeminal nerve are primary sensory neurones with peripheral processes distributed via the ophthalmic, maxillary and mandibular divisions of the

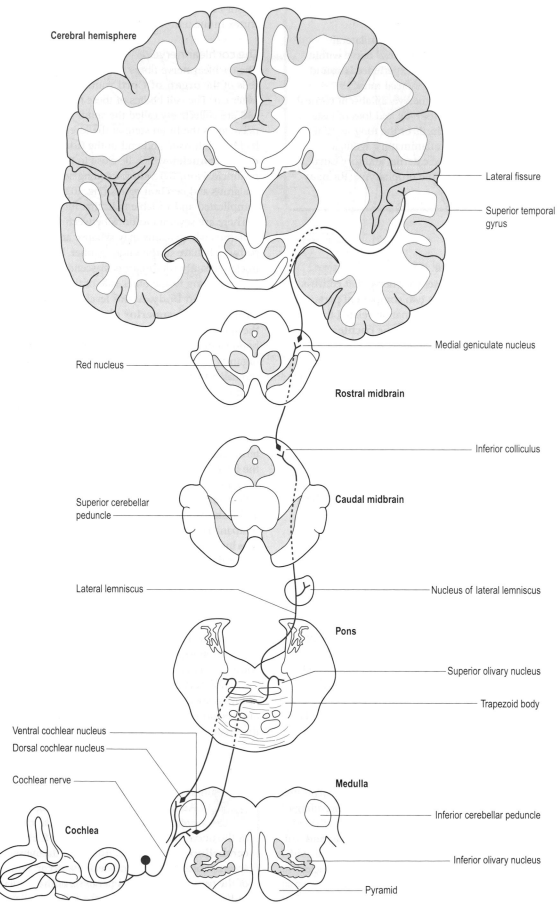

Fig. 10.18 **Principal ascending connections of the auditory component of the vestibulocochlear nerve.**

others do not. The representation of the cochlea is, therefore, essentially bilateral at all levels rostral to the cochlear nuclei. The region of the temporal lobe surrounding the primary auditory cortex is known as the **auditory association cortex** or **Wernicke's area**. It is here that auditory information is interpreted and given contextual significance. Wernicke's area is important in the processing of language by the brain (Chapter 13).

IX: Glossopharyngeal nerve

The glossopharyngeal nerve is principally a sensory nerve, although it also contains preganglionic parasympathetic and a few motor fibres. It attaches to the brain stem as a linear series of small rootlets, lateral to the olive in the rostral medulla (Figs 10.11 and 10.19).

The afferent fibres of the glossopharyngeal nerve convey information from:

- receptors for general sensation in the pharynx, the posterior third of the tongue, Eustachian tube and middle ear
- taste buds of the pharynx and the posterior third of the tongue
- chemoreceptors in the carotid body and baroreceptors in the carotid sinus.

Within the brain stem, afferent fibres for general sensation end in the trigeminal sensory nucleus. Fibres carrying touch information from the pharynx and back of the tongue are important for mediating the **gag reflex**, through

connections with the nucleus ambiguus and the hypoglossal nucleus. Visceral and taste fibres of the glossopharyngeal nerve terminate in the nucleus solitarius of the medulla.

The motor component of the glossopharyngeal nerve is very small. It arises from cells in the rostral part of the nucleus ambiguus of the medulla and innervates just one muscle, the stylopharyngeus, which is involved in swallowing.

Preganglionic parasympathetic fibres in the glossopharyngeal nerve originate in the inferior salivatory nucleus of the rostral medulla. These synapse with postganglionic neurones in the otic ganglion, which in turn innervate the parotid salivary gland.

X: Vagus nerve

Rootlets of the vagus nerve attach to the lateral aspect of the medulla immediately caudal to the glossopharyngeal nerve (Fig. 10.19). The vagus contains afferent, motor and parasympathetic fibres.

The afferent fibres of the vagus convey information from:

- receptors for general sensation in the pharynx, larynx, oesophagus, tympanic membrane, external auditory meatus and part of the concha of the external ear
- chemoreceptors in the aortic bodies and baroreceptors in the aortic arch
- receptors widely distributed throughout the thoracic and abdominal viscera.

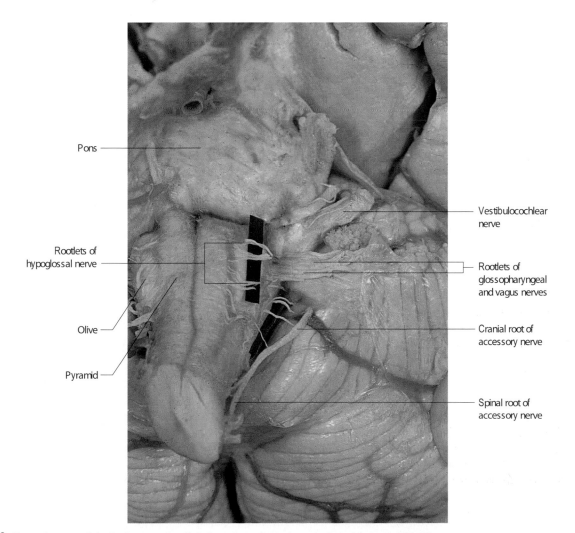

Fig. 10.19 **Ventral aspect of the brain stem showing the points of attachment of cranial nerves VIII–XII.**

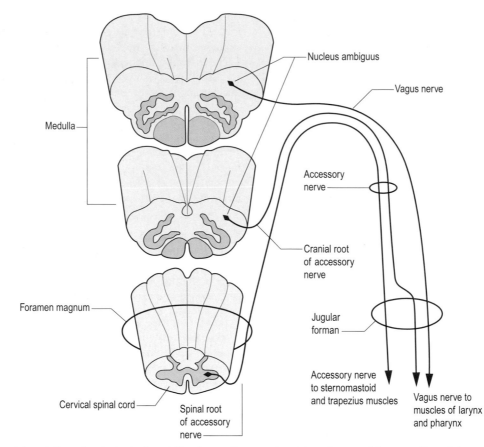

Fig. 10.20 **The caudal medulla and rostral spinal cord.** The diagram illustrates the origin and course of the motor fibres of the vagus and accessory nerves.

Within the brain stem, receptors for general sensation end in the trigeminal sensory nucleus, whilst visceral afferents end in the nucleus solitarius.

The motor fibres of the vagus (Fig. 10.20) arise from the nucleus ambiguus of the medulla. They innervate the muscles of the soft palate, pharynx, larynx and upper part of the oesophagus. The nucleus ambiguus is, therefore, crucially important in the control of speech and swallowing. By convention, the most caudal efferents from the nucleus ambiguus are regarded as leaving the brain stem in the cranial roots of the accessory nerve, but these transfer to the vagus nerve proper at the level of the jugular foramen (Fig. 10.20).

The parasympathetic fibres of the vagus nerve originate from the dorsal motor nucleus of the vagus, which lies in the medulla immediately beneath the floor of the fourth ventricle. They are distributed widely throughout the cardiovascular, respiratory and gastrointestinal systems.

XI: Accessory nerve

The accessory nerve is purely motor in function. It consists of two parts: cranial and spinal. The cranial part emerges from the lateral aspect of the medulla as a linear series of rootlets that lie immediately caudal to the rootlets of the vagus nerve (Figs 10.19 and 10.20). The cranial root of the accessory nerve carries fibres that have their origin in the caudal part of the nucleus ambiguus of the medulla. At the level of the jugular foramen these fibres join the vagus nerve and are distributed with it to the muscles of the soft palate, pharynx and larynx.

The spinal root of the accessory nerve arises from motor neurones located in the ventral horn of the spinal grey matter at levels C1–C5 (Fig. 10.20). The axons leave the cord not through the ventral roots of spinal nerves but via a series of rootlets that emerge from the lateral aspect of the cord midway between the dorsal and ventral roots. These rootlets course rostrally, coalescing as they do so, and enter the cranial cavity through the foramen magnum. At the side of the medulla, the spinal root of the accessory nerve briefly joins the cranial root, but the component fibres separate once again as the nerve leaves the cranial cavity through the jugular foramen. Here the fibres of the cranial root of the accessory, which are derived from the nucleus ambiguus, join the vagus and are distributed with it. The fibres of the spinal root pass to the sternomastoid and trapezius muscles, which serve to move the head and shoulders.

XII: Hypoglossal nerve

The hypoglossal nerve is purely motor in function. It innervates both the extrinsic and intrinsic muscles of the tongue and, therefore, serves both to move and to change the shape of the tongue. The axons originate in the hypoglossal nucleus, which lies immediately beneath the floor of the fourth ventricle, near the midline (Fig. 10.21). Axons course ventrally through the medulla and emerge from its ventrolateral aspect as a linear series of rootlets located between the pyramid and the olive (Fig. 10.19). The hypoglossal nucleus receives afferents from the nucleus solitarius and the trigeminal sensory nucleus. These are involved in the control of the reflex movements of chewing, sucking and swallowing. It also receives corticobulbar fibres from the contralateral motor cortex, which subserve voluntary movements of the tongue such as occur in speech.

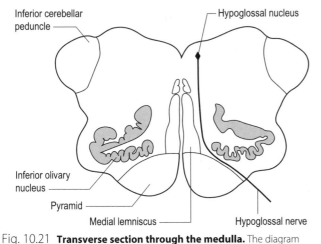

Fig. 10.21 Transverse section through the medulla. The diagram shows the origin and course of the fibres of the hypoglossal nerve.

Inferior cerebellar peduncle
Hypoglossal nucleus
Inferior olivary nucleus
Pyramid
Medial lemniscus
Hypoglossal nerve

Motor neurone disease and lesions of cranial nerves IX–XII

Motor neurone disease is a chronic degenerative disorder seen in those aged over 50 years. The corticobulbar tracts projecting to the nucleus ambiguus and hypoglossal nucleus degenerate, leading to dysphonia (difficulty in phonation), dysphagia (difficulty in swallowing), dysarthria (difficulty in articulation) and weakness and spasticity of the tongue (**pseudobulbar palsy**). There is also degeneration of the nucleus ambiguus and hypoglossal nuclei themselves, leading to dysphonia, dysphagia, dysarthria and weakness, wasting and fasciculation of the tongue (**bulbar palsy**).

The IX, X, XI and XII nerves can be damaged by compression in their peripheral course as they exit the cranium via the foramina of the skull base. Tumours in this area lead to dysphonia, unilateral weakness, wasting and fasciculation of the tongue and depression of the gag reflex, together with unilateral wasting of the sternomastoid and trapezius muscles.

Table 10.1 **Cranial nerves**

Cranial nerve	Component fibres	Structures innervated	Functions
I Olfactory	Sensory	Olfactory epithelium via olfactory bulb	Olfaction
II Optic	Sensory	Retina	Vision
III Oculomotor	Motor	Superior, inferior and medial rectus, inferior oblique, levator palpebrae muscles	Movement of the eyeball
	Parasympathetic	Pupillary constrictor and ciliary muscle of the eyeball, via ciliary ganglion	Pupillary constriction and accommodation
IV Trochlear	Motor	Superior oblique muscle	Movement of the eyeball
V Trigeminal	Sensory	Face, scalp, cornea, nasal and oral cavities, cranial dura mater	General sensation
	Motor	Muscles of mastication	Opening and closing the mouth
		Tensor tympani muscle	Tension on tympanic membrane
VI Abducens	Motor	Lateral rectus muscle	Movement of the eyeball
VII Facial	Sensory	Anterior two-thirds of tongue	Taste
	Motor	Muscles of facial expression	Facial movement
		Stapedius muscle	Tension on bones of middle ear
	Parasympathetic	Salivary and lacrimal glands via submandibular and pterygopalatine ganglia	Salivation and lacrimation
VIII Vestibulocochlear	Sensory	Vestibular apparatus	Vestibular sensation (position and movement of head)
		Cochlea	Hearing
IX Glossopharyngeal	Sensory	Pharynx, posterior third of tongue	General sensation and taste
		Eustachian tube, middle ear	General sensation
		Carotid body and carotid sinus	Chemo- and baroreception
	Motor	Stylopharyngeus muscle	Swallowing
	Parasympathetic	Parotid salivary gland via otic ganglion	Salivation
X Vagus	Sensory	Pharynx, larynx, oesophagus, external ear	General sensation
		Aortic bodies, aortic arch	Chemo- and baroreception
		Thoracic and abdominal viscera	Visceral sensation
	Motor	Soft palate, pharynx, larynx, upper oesophagus	Speech, swallowing
	Parasympathetic	Thoracic and abdominal viscera	Control of cardiovascular system, respiratory and gastrointestinal tracts
XI Accessory	Motor	Sternomastoid and trapezius muscles	Movement of head and shoulder
XII Hypoglossal	Motor	Intrinsic and extrinsic muscles of the tongue	Movement of the tongue

Chapter 11
Cerebellum

The cerebellum is the largest part of the hindbrain. It originates from the dorsal aspect of the brain stem and overlies the fourth ventricle. The cerebellum is connected to the brain stem by three stout pairs of fibre bundles, called the **inferior**, **middle** and **superior cerebellar peduncles** (Fig. 11.1); these join the cerebellum to the medulla, pons and midbrain, respectively. The functions of the cerebellum are entirely motor and it operates at an unconscious level. It controls the maintenance of equilibrium (balance), influences posture and muscle tone, and coordinates movement.

External features of the cerebellum

The cerebellum consists of two laterally located **hemispheres**, joined in the midline by the **vermis** (Figs 11.2–11.4). The superior surface of the cerebellum lies beneath the tentorium cerebelli and the superior vermis is raised, forming a midline ridge. Conversely, the inferior vermis lies in a deep groove between the hemispheres. The surface of the cerebellum is highly convoluted, the folds, or **folia**, being oriented approximately transversely. Between the folia lie fissures of varying depths. Some of these fissures are landmarks that are used to divide the cerebellum anatomically into three lobes (Figs 11.2–11.5). On the superior surface, the deep **primary fissure** separates the relatively small **anterior lobe** from the much larger **posterior lobe**. On the underside, the conspicuous **posterolateral fissure** demarcates the location of small regions of the hemisphere (the **flocculus**) and vermis (the **nodule**), which together form the **flocculonodular lobe**.

External features of the cerebellum

- The cerebellum controls the maintenance of equilibrium, posture and muscle tone and it coordinates movement. It operates at an unconscious level.
- The cerebellum is connected to the medulla, pons and midbrain by the inferior, middle and superior cerebellar peduncles, respectively.
- The cerebellum consists of a midline vermis and two laterally located hemispheres.
- Anatomically, the cerebellum is divided into anterior, posterior and flocculonodular lobes.

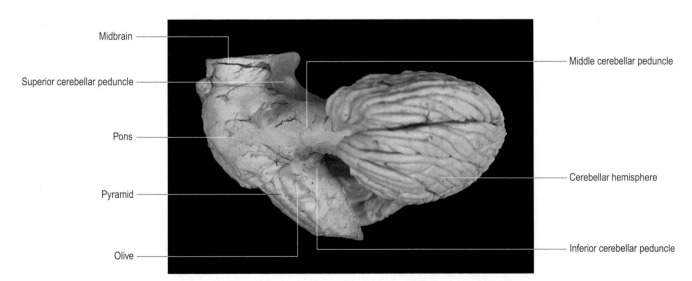

Fig. 11.1 **Lateral aspect of the brain stem and cerebellum, showing the cerebellar peduncles.** Parts of the anterior, posterior and flocculonodular lobes have been removed to display the peduncles more clearly.

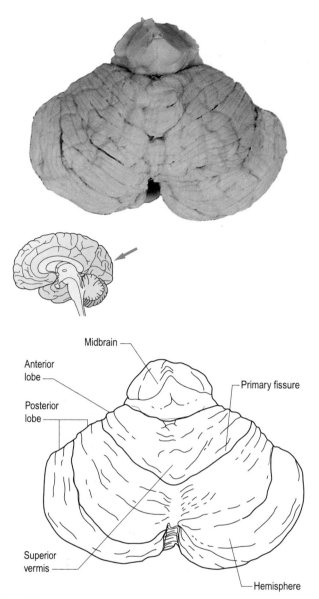

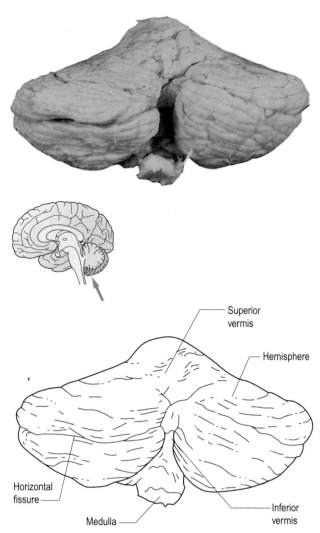

Fig. 11.2 **Superior surface of the cerebellum.**

Labels for Fig. 11.2:
- Midbrain
- Anterior lobe
- Posterior lobe
- Primary fissure
- Superior vermis
- Hemisphere

Fig. 11.3 **Posterior aspect of the cerebellum.**

Labels for Fig. 11.3:
- Superior vermis
- Hemisphere
- Horizontal fissure
- Medulla
- Inferior vermis

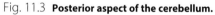

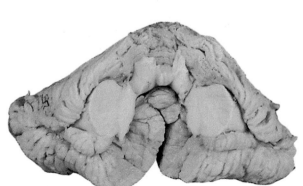

Fig. 11.4 **Anteroinferior aspect of the cerebellum.**

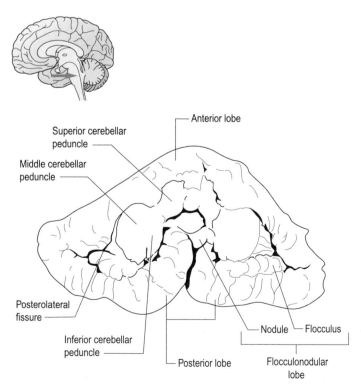

Labels for Fig. 11.4:
- Anterior lobe
- Superior cerebellar peduncle
- Middle cerebellar peduncle
- Posterolateral fissure
- Inferior cerebellar peduncle
- Posterior lobe
- Nodule
- Flocculus
- Flocculonodular lobe

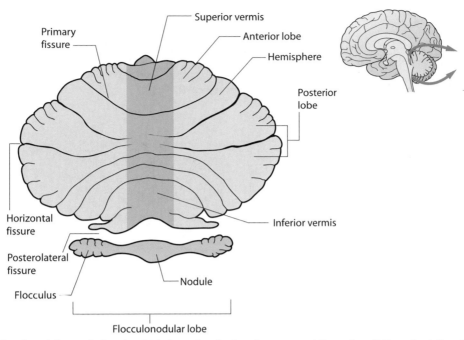

Fig. 11.5 **Schematic drawing of the cerebellum in which the peduncles have been cut and the surface flattened out.** The relationships between the anatomical and functional divisions of the cerebellum are shown. (Green, archicerebellum; blue, paleocerebellum; pink, neocerebellum.)

Internal structure of the cerebellum

The cerebellum basically consists of an outer layer of grey matter, the **cerebellar cortex**, and an inner core of white matter. The white matter is made up largely of afferent and efferent fibres that run to and from the cortex and towards which it extends irregular, branch-like projections (Fig. 11.6). Buried deep within the white matter are four pairs of **cerebellar nuclei** (Figs 11.6 and 11.7), which have important connections with the cerebellar cortex and with certain nuclei of the brain stem and thalamus.

Cerebellar cortex

The cerebellar cortex is highly convoluted, forming numerous transversely oriented folia. Within the cortex lie the cell bodies, dendrites and synaptic connections of the vast majority of cerebellar neurones. The cellular organisation of the cortex is the same in all regions (Fig. 11.8). It is divided histologically into three layers:

- the outer, fibre-rich, **molecular layer**
- the intermediate, **Purkinje cell layer**
- the inner **granular layer**, which is dominated by the **granule cell**.

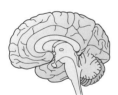

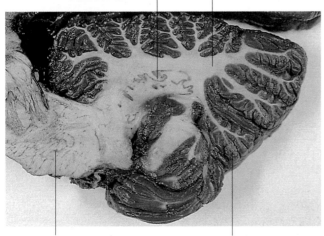

Fig. 11.6 **Parasagittal section through the cerebellum.** Mulligan's stain.

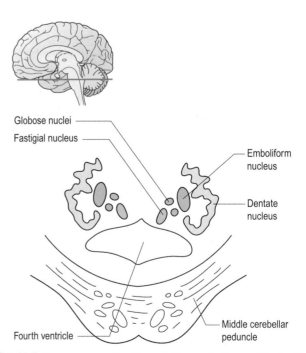

Fig. 11.7 **Transverse section through the cerebellum and brain stem at the level of the fourth ventricle, showing the cerebellar nuclei.**

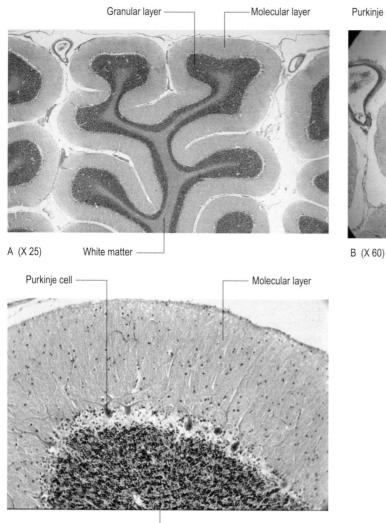

Granular layer — — Molecular layer

A (X 25)   White matter —

Purkinje cell layer — — Molecular layer

B (X 60)   White matter — — Granular layer

Purkinje cell — — Molecular layer

C (X 160)   — Granular layer

Fig. 11.8 **Transverse sections of cerebellar folia showing the layers of the cerebellar cortex.**

Afferent projections to the cerebellum arise principally from the spinal cord (spinocerebellar fibres), inferior olivary nucleus (olivocerebellar fibres), vestibular nuclei (vestibulocerebellar fibres) and pons (pontocerebellar fibres). Afferent axons mostly terminate in the cerebellar cortex, where they are excitatory to cortical neurones. Fibres enter the cerebellum through one of the cerebellar peduncles and proceed to the cortex as either **mossy fibres** or **climbing fibres**, depending upon their origin (Fig. 11.9). All afferents originating elsewhere than the inferior olivary nucleus end as mossy fibres. Mossy fibres branch to supply several folia and end in the granular layer, in synaptic contact with granule cells. The axons of granule cells pass towards the surface of the cortex and enter the molecular layer. Here they bifurcate to produce two **parallel fibres** that are oriented along the long axis of the folium.

The Purkinje cell layer consists of a unicellular layer of the somata of Purkinje neurones. The profuse dendritic arborisations of these cells (see Fig. 2.1B) extend towards the surface of the cortex, into the molecular layer (Fig. 11.9). The arborisations are flattened and oriented at right angles to the long axis of the folium. They are, therefore, traversed by numerous parallel fibres, from which they receive excitatory synaptic input. Inhibitory modulation of intracortical circuitry is provided by numerous other neurones known as

Golgi, basket and stellate cells. The axons of Purkinje cells are the only axons to leave the cerebellar cortex. Most of these fibres do not leave the cerebellum entirely but end in the deep cerebellar nuclei. The other type of afferent fibre entering the cerebellar cortex, the climbing fibre, originates from the inferior olivary nucleus of the medulla. These fibres provide relatively discrete excitatory input to Purkinje cells. At the same time, axon collaterals of climbing fibres excite the neurones of the deep cerebellar nuclei. Purkinje cells utilise GABA as their neurotransmitter, which means that the output of almost the whole of the cerebellar cortex is mediated through the inhibition of cells in the cerebellar nuclei.

Cerebellar nuclei

Deep within the cerebellar white matter, above the roof of the fourth ventricle, lie four pairs of nuclei. From medial to lateral, they are known as:

- fastigial nucleus
- globose nucleus
- emboliform nucleus
- dentate nucleus (Figs 11.6 and 11.7).

The dentate nucleus is by far the largest of the cerebellar nuclei and is the only one that can be discerned clearly with

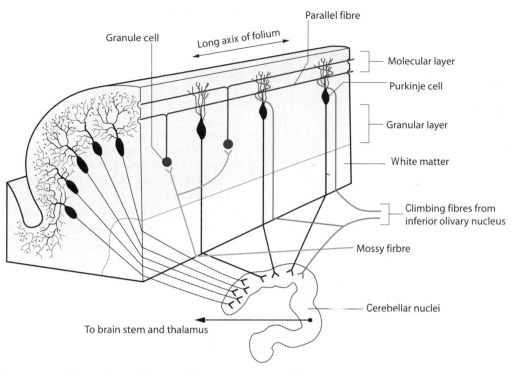

Fig. 11.9 **The cerebellar cortex.** Diagram shows afferent and efferent connections and their relationships to the principal cells of the cerebellar cortex.

Internal structure of the cerebellum

- Internally, the cerebellum consists of a surface layer of cortex, highly convoluted to form folia, beneath which lies white matter.
- Within the white matter lie cerebellar nuclei (fastigial, globose, emboliform and dentate).
- The nuclei are the origin of cerebellar efferent fibres.

the naked eye (Fig. 11.6). It consists of a thin layer of nerve cells folded into a crinkled bag; as a result, it appears somewhat similar to the inferior olivary nucleus of the medulla, from which it receives afferent fibres. The cerebellar nuclei also receive extracerebellar afferents from the vestibular nuclei, reticular nuclei, pontine nuclei and spinocerebellar tracts, predominantly by means of collaterals of mossy fibres destined for the cerebellar cortex. From within the cerebellum, the nuclei receive dense innervation from the Purkinje cells of the cerebellar cortex itself. The cerebellar nuclei constitute the primary source of efferent fibres from the cerebellum to other parts of the brain. The principal destinations of efferent fibres are the reticular and vestibular nuclei of the medulla and pons, the red nucleus of the midbrain and the ventral lateral nucleus of the thalamus.

Functional anatomy of the cerebellum

The cerebellum is often regarded as consisting of three functional subdivisions, based upon phylogenetic, anatomical and functional considerations (Fig. 11.5).

- The **archicerebellum**, or oldest portion in phylogenetic terms, is equated with the **flocculonodular lobe** and the associated **fastigial** nuclei.

- The **paleocerebellum** approximates to the midline **vermis** and surrounding **paravermis**, together with the **globose** and **emboliform** nuclei.
- The **neocerebellum** comprises the remainder (and vast majority) of the **cerebellar hemisphere** and the **dentate nuclei**.

Archicerebellum

The archicerebellum is primarily concerned with the maintenance of balance (equilibrium). It has extensive connections with the vestibular and reticular nuclei of the brain stem, through the inferior cerebellar peduncles (Fig. 11.10). Vestibular information is carried from the vestibular nuclei to the cortex of the ipsilateral flocculonodular lobe. Cortical efferent (Purkinje cell) fibres project to the fastigial nucleus, which, in turn, projects back to the vestibular nuclei and to the reticular formation. A significant proportion of fastigial efferents cross to the contralateral side of the brain stem. The influence of the archicerebellum upon the lower motor system is, therefore, bilateral and principally mediated by means of descending vestibulospinal and reticulospinal projections.

Paleocerebellum

The paleocerebellum influences muscle tone and posture. Afferents consist principally of dorsal and ventral spinocerebellar tract neurones that carry information from muscle, joint and cutaneous receptors and enter the cerebellum through the inferior and superior cerebellar peduncles, respectively (Fig. 11.11). Fibres terminate largely in the cortex of the ipsilateral vermis and paravermis. Cerebellar cortical efferents from these areas pass to the globose and emboliform nuclei and also to the fastigial nucleus. The globose and emboliform nuclei project via the superior cerebellar peduncle to the contralateral red nucleus of the midbrain, where they influence the activity of cells giving rise to the descending rubrospinal tract.

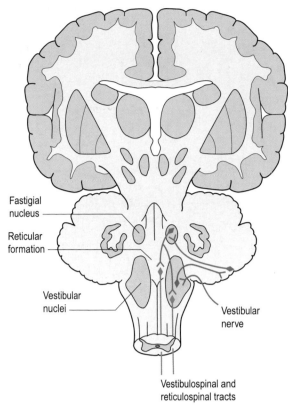

Fastigial nucleus

Reticular formation

Vestibular nuclei

Vestibular nerve

Vestibulospinal and reticulospinal tracts

Fig. 11.10 **Connections of the archicerebellum.** Contralateral projections of the fastigial nucleus are not shown.

Neocerebellum

The neocerebellum is concerned with muscular coordination, including the trajectory, speed and force of movements. The principal afferent pathway consists of pontocerebellar fibres (Fig. 11.12). These originate in the pontine nuclei of the basal portion of the pons and cross to the opposite side, entering the cerebellum through its middle peduncle. Pontocerebellar neurones are influenced by widespread regions of the cerebral cortex involved in the planning and execution of movement. Pontocerebellar fibres terminate predominantly in the lateral parts of the cerebellar hemisphere. Output from the neocerebellar cortex is directed to the dentate nucleus. The dentate nucleus, in turn, projects to the contralateral red nucleus and ventral lateral nucleus of the thalamus. The dentate is the largest of the cerebellar nuclei and its efferents form a major part of the superior cerebellar peduncle. The fibres decussate in the caudal midbrain just before reaching the red nucleus. Some relay in the red nucleus with rubrothalamic cells but most bypass the red nucleus and pass directly to the ventral lateral thalamus. The ventral lateral nucleus of the thalamus projects to the cerebral cortex, particularly the motor cortex of the frontal lobe. The neocerebellum thus exerts its coordinating role in movement primarily through an action on cerebral cortical areas, giving rise to descending corticospinal and corticobulbar pathways.

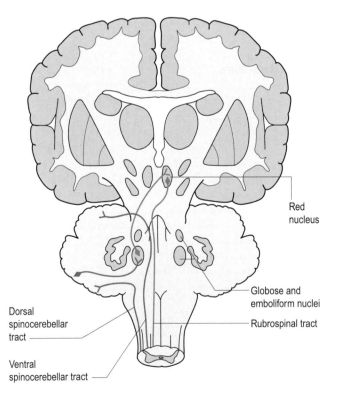

Red nucleus

Globose and emboliform nuclei

Rubrospinal tract

Dorsal spinocerebellar tract

Ventral spinocerebellar tract

Fig. 11.11 **Connections of the paleocerebellum.**

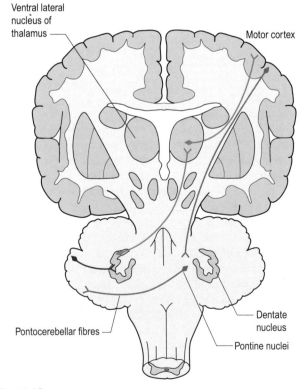

Ventral lateral nucleus of thalamus

Motor cortex

Pontocerebellar fibres

Dentate nucleus

Pontine nuclei

Fig. 11.12 **Connections of the neocerebellum.**

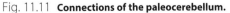

Lesions of the cerebellum

A midline lesion of the cerebellum (such as a tumour) leads to loss of postural control; as a result it is impossible to stand or sit without toppling over, despite preserved coordination of the limbs.

Because of the pattern of ipsilateral and decussated pathways that enter and leave the cerebellum, unilateral lesions of the cerebellar hemisphere cause symptoms on the same side of the body. This is in contrast to cerebral lesions (e.g. in the cerebral cortex, internal capsule or basal ganglia), which give rise to contralateral symptoms.

A unilateral cerebellar hemispheric lesion causes ipsilateral incoordination of the arm (**intention tremor**) and of the leg, causing an unsteady gait, in the absence of weakness or sensory loss.

Bilateral dysfunction of the cerebellum, caused by alcoholic intoxication, hypothyroidism, inherited cerebellar degeneration/ataxia, multiple sclerosis or paraneoplastic disease, causes slowness and slurring of speech (**dysarthria**), incoordination of both arms and a staggering, wide-based, unsteady gait (**cerebellar ataxia**).

Cerebellar lesions also impair coordination of eye movements and the eyes exhibit a to-and-fro motion (**nystagmus**), greatest in amplitude when gaze is directed to the same side as the lesion. Nystagmus is a very common feature of multiple sclerosis. The combination of nystagmus with dysarthria and intention tremor constitutes '**Charcot's triad**', which is highly diagnostic of the disease.

Functional anatomy of the cerebellum

- The archicerebellum corresponds to the flocculonodular lobe and fastigial nucleus. Its principal connections are with the vestibular and reticular nuclei of the brain stem and it is concerned with the maintenance of equilibrium.
- The paleocerebellum corresponds to the vermis and paravermal area, together with the globose and emboliform nuclei. It receives fibres from the spinocerebellar tracts and projects to the red nucleus of the midbrain.
- The neocerebellum corresponds to most of the cerebellar hemisphere and the dentate nucleus. It receives afferents from the pons and projects to the ventral lateral nucleus of the thalamus.
- Cerebellar lesions cause incoordination of the upper limbs (intention tremor), lower limbs (cerebellar ataxia), speech (dysarthria) and eyes (nystagmus).

Chapter 12
Thalamus

Rostral to the midbrain lies the forebrain (prosencephalon, cerebrum; Fig. 1.10). The forebrain consists of the bilaterally paired diencephalon and cerebral hemisphere on each side and is by far the largest derivative of the three basic embryological divisions of the brain. The diencephalon is continuous with the rostral part of the midbrain and lies between the brain stem and the cerebral hemisphere. The diencephalon comprises, from dorsal to ventral: the epithalamus, thalamus, subthalamus and hypothalamus, of which the thalamus is the largest. The thalamus consists of numerous nuclei, most of which have extensive reciprocal connections with the cerebral cortex. Of particular note are:

- nuclei that transmit general and special sensory information to corresponding regions of the sensory cortices
- nuclei that receive impulses from the cerebellum and basal ganglia and interface with motor regions of the frontal lobe

- nuclei that have connections with associative and limbic areas of the cortex.

The diencephalon is almost entirely surrounded by the cerebral hemisphere; consequently, little of its structure can be seen externally, apart from the ventral portion of the hypothalamus, which can be seen on the base of the brain (Fig. 12.1). Immediately caudal to the optic chiasma is a small midline elevation, the **tuber cinereum**. From its apex extends the **infundibulum** or pituitary stalk, which attaches to the pituitary gland. Caudal to the tuber cinereum, a pair of rounded eminences, the **mammillary bodies**, are located on either side of the midline. These contain the mammillary nuclei of the **hypothalamus**. The hypothalamus lies below the thalamus, extending medial and ventral to the subthalamus. It has important connections with the limbic system, a controlling influence upon the activity of the autonomic nervous system and a central role in neuroendocrine function, partly through its relationship with the pituitary gland. The hypothalamus is discussed further in Chapter 16.

The other parts of the diencephalon can be seen in sagittal and coronal sections of the brain (Figs 12.2 and 12.3). The diencephalon forms the lateral wall of the third ventricle. The dorsal part of the ventricular wall is formed by the thalamus and the ventral part by the hypothalamus. The **epithalamus** is a relatively small part of the diencephalon located in its most caudal and dorsal region, immediately rostral to the superior colliculus of the midbrain. It consists principally of the **pineal gland** and the **habenular nuclei**.

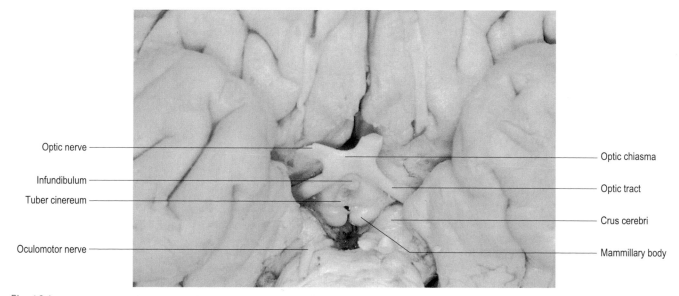

Optic nerve — Infundibulum — Tuber cinereum — Oculomotor nerve — Optic chiasma — Optic tract — Crus cerebri — Mammillary body

Fig. 12.1 **Ventral aspect of the diencephalon.**

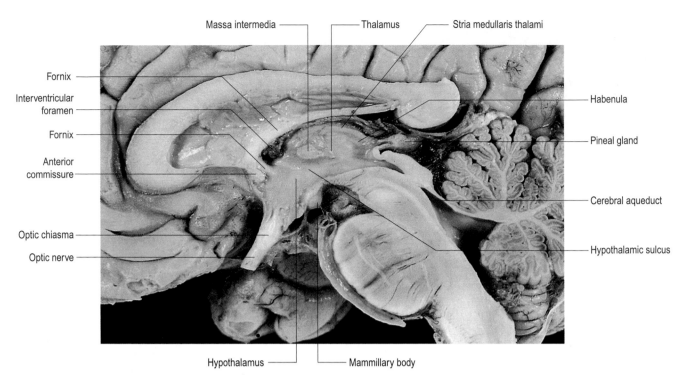

Fig. 12.2 **Median sagittal section of the brain showing the relationships of the diencephalon.**

The pineal gland is an endocrine organ. It synthesises the hormone melatonin. The pineal gland has been implicated in control of the sleep/waking cycle (circadian rhythm) and in regulation of the onset of puberty. The habenular nuclei have connections with the limbic system (Chapter 16).

The **subthalamus** lies beneath the thalamus and dorsolateral to the hypothalamus, with its ventrolateral aspect against the internal capsule. It contains two notable cell groups, the subthalamic nucleus and the zona incerta. The subthalamic nucleus is located in the ventrolateral part of the subthalamus, immediately medial to the internal capsule. It has the shape of a biconvex lens in coronal section. The subthalamic nucleus has prominent connections with the globus pallidus and the substantia nigra and is important in the control of movement. It is discussed in more detail in Chapter 14. The zona incerta is a rostral extension of the brain stem reticular formation. Several important fibre systems traverse the subthalamus en route to the thalamus. These include ascending sensory projections (medial lemniscus, spinothalamic tracts, trigeminothalamic tracts), cerebellothalamic fibres from the dentate nucleus and pallidothalamic fibres from the medial segment of the globus pallidus. The last envelop the zona incerta as the lenticular fasciculus and thalamic fasciculus.

Topographical anatomy of the thalamus

External features

The thalamus has been likened in size and shape to a small hen's egg. Together with the hypothalamus it forms the lateral wall of the third ventricle, the transition between the two being marked by a faint groove, the hypothalamic sulcus. In most individuals, the two thalami are joined across the thin slit of the ventricle by the **interthalamic adhesion** or **massa intermedia**. A fascicle of nerve fibres, the **stria medullaris**, which has limbic connections, courses along the dorsomedial margin of the thalamus (Fig. 12.2). Along this line, the ependymal lining of the third ventricle spans the narrow lumen to form the ventricular roof.

The anterior pole of the thalamus extends as far as the interventricular foramen, through which the third and lateral ventricles are in continuity. Lateral to the thalamus lies the posterior limb of the internal capsule and anterolateral lies the head of the caudate nucleus (Fig. 12.4). The dorsal aspect of the thalamus thus forms part of the floor of the body of the lateral ventricle. Another fascicle of nerve fibres with limbic connections, the **stria terminalis**, marks the boundary between thalamus and caudate (Fig. 12.4). Ventral to the thalamus lie the subthalamus and hypothalamus; caudal to it lies the midbrain.

Internal organisation

Within the thalamus is located a thin layer of nerve fibres composed of some of the afferent and efferent connections of thalamic nuclei. This is called the **internal medullary lamina** (Figs 12.3, 12.5 and 12.6). The lamina is roughly Y-shaped when viewed from above and provides the basis

---

Anatomy of the thalamus

- The thalamus is the largest component of the diencephalon, which is situated between the brain stem and the cerebral hemisphere.
- Almost all thalamic nuclei have rich reciprocal connections with the cerebral cortex.
- The thalamus is divided into three principal nuclear masses (anterior, medial and lateral) by the internal medullary lamina.
- Embedded within the internal medullary lamina lie intralaminar nuclei.
- On the lateral aspect of the thalamus lies the thin reticular nucleus.

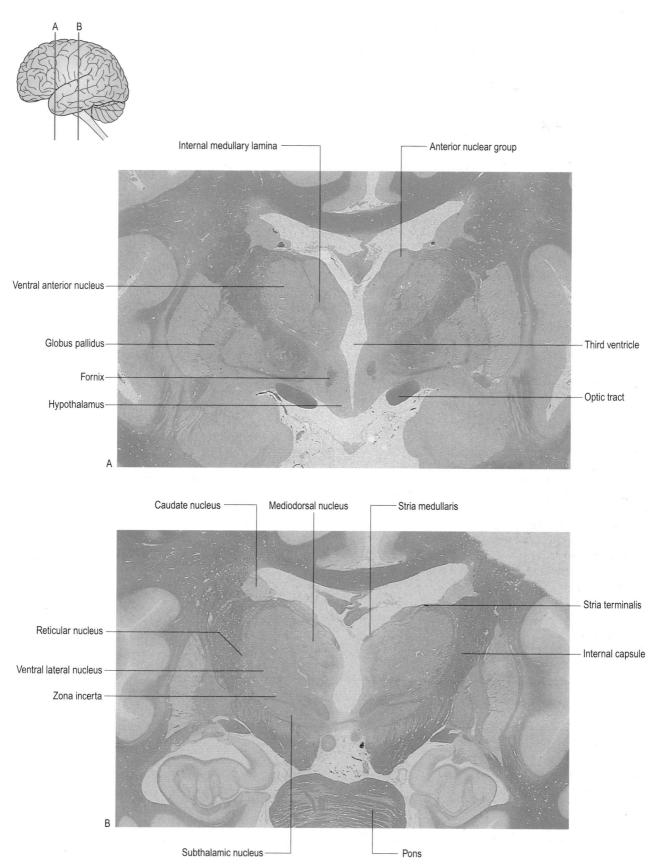

Fig. 12.3 **Coronal sections through the diencephalon.** Luxol fast blue stain for myelin.

for dividing the main part of the thalamus into three nuclear masses: **anterior**, **medial** and **lateral**. Each of these cellular complexes is further subdivided into a number of individually named nuclei. Embedded within the internal medullary lamina are several cell groups, known collectively as the **intralaminar nuclei** (Fig. 12.6). Lateral to the main

mass of thalamic nuclei lies another sheet of nerve fibres, the **lateral medullary lamina**, which consists of thalamocortical and corticothalamic fibres. Between this and the internal capsule is located a thin stratum of neurones that constitute the **reticular nucleus** of the thalamus (Fig. 12.3).

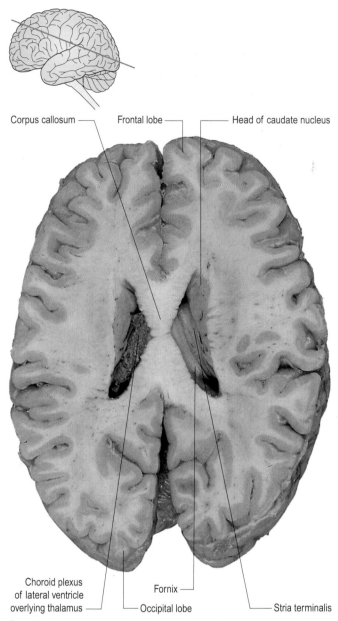

Fig. 12.4 **Dorsal aspect of the diencephalon.** The choroid plexus has been removed on the right side.

Labels: Corpus callosum — Frontal lobe — Head of caudate nucleus; Choroid plexus of lateral ventricle overlying thalamus — Fornix — Occipital lobe — Stria terminalis

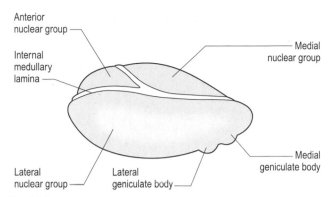

Fig. 12.5 **Dorsolateral view of the left thalamus showing the disposition of the internal medullary lamina and the principal nuclear divisions.**

Labels: Anterior nuclear group; Internal medullary lamina; Lateral nuclear group; Lateral geniculate body; Medial nuclear group; Medial geniculate body

Functional organisation of thalamic nuclei

All the nuclei of the thalamus, with the exception of the reticular nucleus, project to the ipsilateral cerebral cortex and the whole of the cortex receives input from the thalamus. Similarly, all thalamic nuclei receive corticofugal fibres in a basically reciprocal fashion. In some cases, precise, point-to-point projections exist between individual thalamic nuclei and restricted cortical zones with well-defined sensory or motor functions. This typifies the relationship between the thalamic nuclei and cortical regions that subserve the general and special senses and the motor regions that receive cerebellar and basal ganglia input.

Such thalamic nuclei are often referred to as the 'specific' nuclei. The specific nuclei all lie within the ventral part (tier) of the lateral nuclear group. Other thalamic nuclei receive less functionally distinct afferent input that does not include overtly sensory or motor pathways; in turn, these connect with wider areas of cortex, including associative and limbic domains. These are often referred to as the 'non-specific' nuclei. Non-specific thalamic nuclei include the nuclei of the dorsal tier of the lateral nuclear complex as well as the whole of the anterior and medial complexes.

Thalamic lesions

Strokes and tumours destroying the thalamus lead to loss of sensation in the contralateral face and limbs, accompanied by a distressing discomfort in the paradoxically anaesthetic areas (**thalamic pain**). Thalamic lesions may mimic focal cortical defects because of the richness of thalamocortical connections.

Lateral nuclear group

The lateral nuclear group contains all of the so-called 'specific' thalamic nuclei. These are located in the ventral part of the complex and include the ventral anterior, ventral lateral, ventral posterior, lateral geniculate and medial geniculate nuclei (Fig. 12.6).

Ventral posterior nucleus

The ventral posterior (VP) nucleus lies between the ventrolateral nucleus and the pulvinar. Within the ventral posterior nucleus there is termination of all the ascending pathways from the spinal cord and brain stem that carry general sensory information from the contralateral half of the body to a conscious level. These pathways include the spinothalamic tracts, medial lemniscus and trigeminothalamic tracts. The termination of these fibres in the ventral posterior nucleus is highly organised somatotopically.

An extensive, lateral portion of the nucleus receives information from the trunk and limbs via the spinothalamic tracts and medial lemniscus. This is referred to as the ventral posterolateral (VPl) division. A smaller, medial portion of the ventral posterior nucleus receives information from the head, via the trigeminothalamic tract, and is termed the ventral posteromedial nucleus (VPm). This area also receives taste information from the nucleus solitarius of the medulla and vestibular information from the vestibular nuclei. The ventral posterior nucleus projects to the primary somatosensory cortex in the postcentral gyrus of the parietal lobe.

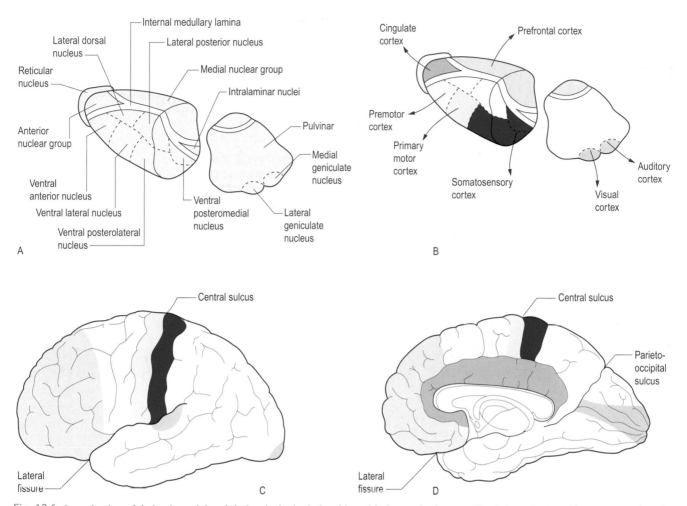

Fig. 12.6 **Organisation of thalamic nuclei and their principal relationships with the cerebral cortex.** The thalamus is viewed from its posterolateral aspect. The posterior part has been sectioned from the rest to reveal the internal structure. In **(A)** the principal thalamic nuclei are identified and in **(B)** their efferent connections are indicated. Colours represent the interrelationships between thalamic nuclei and cerebral cortical regions on the lateral **(C)** and medial **(D)** aspects of the cerebral hemisphere.

Lateral geniculate nucleus

The geniculate nuclei are located near the posterior pole of the thalamus, ventral to the pulvinar. Here they form small eminences on the surface, known as the geniculate bodies. The lateral geniculate nucleus is a part of the visual system and receives further discussion in Chapter 15. It is the site of termination of the optic tract, which carries the axons of retinal ganglion cells. As a result of hemidecussation of optic nerve fibres in the optic chiasma, each nucleus receives axons that have originated in the ipsilateral temporal hemiretina and the contralateral nasal hemiretina and is thus provided with visual information relating to the contralateral half of the visual field. The lateral geniculate nucleus sends fibres, via the retrolenticular part of the internal capsule and the optic radiation, to the primary visual cortex of the occipital lobe.

Medial geniculate nucleus

The medial geniculate nucleus is part of the auditory system, which is described in Chapter 10. It receives ascending fibres from the inferior colliculus of the midbrain, via the inferior brachium. The medial geniculate nucleus projects, via the retrolenticular part of the internal capsule and the auditory radiation, to the primary auditory cortex of the temporal lobe.

Ventral anterior nucleus

The ventral anterior (VA) nucleus occupies the rostral part of the lateral nuclear mass. It consists of two subdivisions: the larger, principal part (VApc) and the smaller, magnocellular part (VAmc). The principal subcortical afferents to this region are output fibres of the ipsilateral basal ganglia system, which originate from the medial segment of the globus pallidus and its homologue, the pars reticulata of the substantia nigra. Fibres from the globus pallidus terminate in VApc, while those from the substantia nigra end in VAmc. The ventral anterior nucleus of the thalamus has reciprocal connections with motor regions of the frontal lobe, particularly the premotor and supplementary motor cortices. It is, therefore, an important part of the mechanism by which the basal ganglia exert their influence on normal movement and through which abnormalities of movement are mediated in basal ganglia disorders.

Ventral lateral nucleus

The ventral lateral (VL) nucleus lies immediately caudal to the ventral anterior nucleus in the ventral tier of the lateral nuclear complex. It consists of three subdivisions: pars oralis (VLo), pars medialis (VLm) and pars caudalis (VLc). Subcortical afferents to the ventral lateral nucleus originate

Functional organisation of the lateral nuclear group

- 'Specific' thalamic nuclei have well-defined sensory or motor functions and highly organised connections with sensory and motor regions of the cerebral cortex. They all lie within the ventral tier of the lateral nuclear mass and include:
  - Ventral posterior nucleus: receives general sensory afferents in the medial lemniscus, spinothalamic tract and trigeminothalamic tract; sends efferents to the primary somatosensory cortex of the parietal lobe.
  - Lateral geniculate nucleus: receives visual afferents in the optic tract; projects to the primary visual cortex of the occipital lobe.
  - Medial geniculate nucleus: receives auditory afferents from the inferior colliculus; sends efferents to the primary auditory cortex of the temporal lobe.
  - Ventral anterior and ventral lateral nuclei: receive afferents from the cerebellum and basal ganglia; send efferents to motor cortical areas of the frontal lobe.
- 'Non-specific' nuclei connect with wider areas of cortex, including associative and limbic regions.

mainly from the ipsilateral globus pallidus and substantia nigra, and from the contralateral dentate nucleus of the cerebellum. Pallidal and nigral afferents terminate in VLo and VLm, while those from the cerebellum terminate in VLc. The ventral lateral nucleus, like the ventral anterior nucleus, has reciprocal connections with motor areas of the frontal lobe and especially with the primary motor cortex of the precentral gyrus.

Within the dorsal tier of the lateral nuclear complex lie a number of so-called 'non-specific' nuclei. Amongst these, the lateral dorsal nucleus is part of the limbic system. It receives afferents from the hippocampus and sends efferents to the cingulate gyrus. The lateral posterior nucleus has connections with the sensory association cortex of the parietal lobe. The **pulvinar** is a large region at the most posterior part of the thalamus. It has extensive connections with association cortices of the parietal, temporal and occipital lobes.

Anterior nuclear group

The most anterior portion of the thalamus, extending to its rostral pole, is the anterior nuclear complex. It consists of three subdivisions: the anteroventral, anteromedial and anterodorsal nuclei. The individual connections of these will not be discussed. The anterior nuclear group is part of the limbic system. It receives a large afferent projection from the mammillary body of the hypothalamus via the mammillothalamic tract. The anterior complex projects principally to the cingulate gyrus on the medial surface of the cerebral hemisphere. It is involved in the control of instinctive drives, in the emotional aspects of behaviour and in memory.

Medial nuclear group

The medial nuclear group forms a large region consisting primarily of the mediodorsal nucleus (dorsomedial nucleus) and some much smaller components, such as the nucleus reuniens. Subcortical afferents to the mediodorsal nucleus come from the hypothalamus, amygdala and from other thalamic nuclei, including the intralaminar nuclei and nuclei of the lateral complex. Extensive reciprocal connections exist between the mediodorsal nucleus and the prefrontal cortex. It is concerned mainly with the control of mood and the emotions.

Intralaminar nuclei

Several nuclei lie embedded within the internal medullary lamina of the thalamus. These include the centromedian and parafascicular nuclei, the centromedian being the largest intralaminar nucleus in humans. The intralaminar nuclei receive ascending afferents from the brain stem reticular formation and also from the spinothalamic and trigeminothalamic systems. In turn, they project to widespread regions of the cerebral cortex and to the caudate nucleus and putamen of the basal ganglia. The intralaminar nuclei are part of the mechanism for activation of the cerebral cortical mantle. When they are stimulated, alpha rhythm activity, which is associated with repose and sleep, is disrupted and the electroencephalogram (EEG) becomes desynchronised. Lesions of the intralaminar nuclei reduce the perception of pain and the level of consciousness.

Reticular nucleus

The reticular nucleus is a thin layer of cells located on the lateral aspect of the thalamus between the external medullary lamina and the internal capsule. This nucleus receives collaterals of both thalamocortical and corticothalamic fibres, which pass between other thalamic nuclei and the cerebral cortex.

Functional organisation of anterior, medial, intralaminar and reticular nuclei

- The anterior nuclear group of the thalamus is part of the limbic system. This region receives fibres from the mammillary body of the hypothalamus and projects to the cingulate gyrus.
- Within the medial nuclear group, the mediodorsal nucleus has extensive reciprocal connections with the cortex of the frontal lobe.
- The intralaminar nuclei receive input from the reticular formation and ascending sensory systems. They project to the cerebral cortex and the striatum and are responsible for activation of the cerebral cortex.
- The reticular nucleus receives collaterals of thalamocortical and corticothalamic fibres.

Chapter 13
Cerebral hemisphere and cerebral cortex

The cerebral hemisphere is derived from the embryological telencephalon (Chapter 1). It is the largest part of the forebrain and it reaches the greatest degree of development in the human brain. Superficially, the cerebral hemisphere consists of a layer of grey matter, the cerebral cortex, which is highly convoluted to form a complex pattern of ridges (gyri) and furrows (sulci). This serves to maximise the surface area of the cerebral cortex, about 70% of which is hidden within the depths of sulci (Figs 13.1 and 13.2). Beneath the surface, axons running to and from the cells of the cortex form an extensive mass of white matter. Figures 13.3–13.12 show successive coronal sections through the brain. The vast majority of those nerve fibres that pass between the cerebral cortex and subcortical structures are condensed, deep within the hemisphere, into a broad sheet called the **internal capsule** (Figs 13.4–13.11; see also

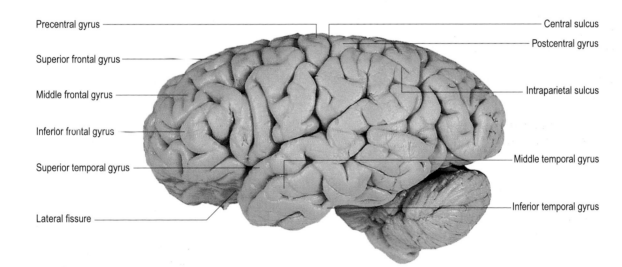

Precentral gyrus — Central sulcus — Postcentral gyrus
Superior frontal gyrus
Middle frontal gyrus — Intraparietal sulcus
Inferior frontal gyrus
Superior temporal gyrus — Middle temporal gyrus
— Inferior temporal gyrus
Lateral fissure

Fig. 13.1 **Lateral aspect of the cerebral hemisphere showing major gyri and sulci.**

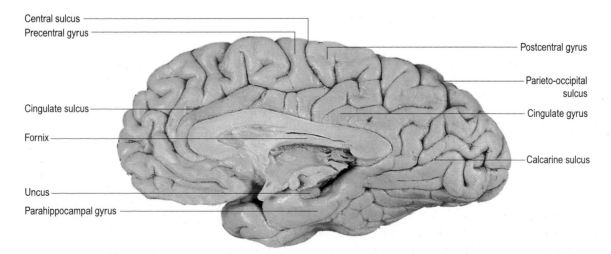

Central sulcus
Precentral gyrus — Postcentral gyrus
— Parieto-occipital sulcus
Cingulate sulcus — Cingulate gyrus
Fornix
— Calcarine sulcus
Uncus
Parahippocampal gyrus

Fig. 13.2 **Median sagittal section of the cerebral hemisphere showing major gyri and sulci.** The brain stem and cerebellum have been removed to show the inferomedial aspect of the temporal lobe.

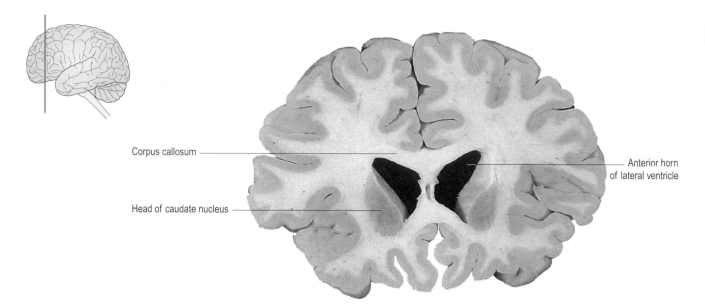

Fig. 13.3 **Coronal section of the cerebral hemisphere.**

Corpus callosum

Anterior horn of lateral ventricle

Head of caudate nucleus

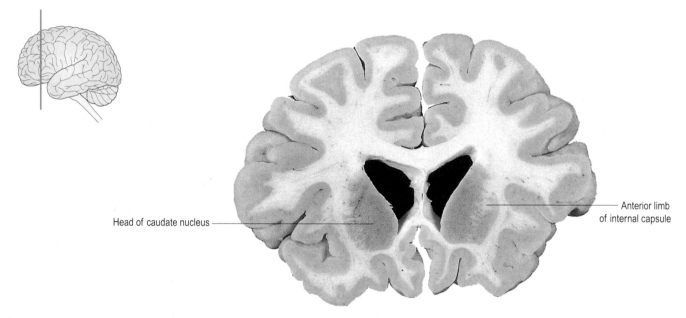

Fig. 13.4 **Coronal section of the cerebral hemisphere.**

Head of caudate nucleus

Anterior limb of internal capsule

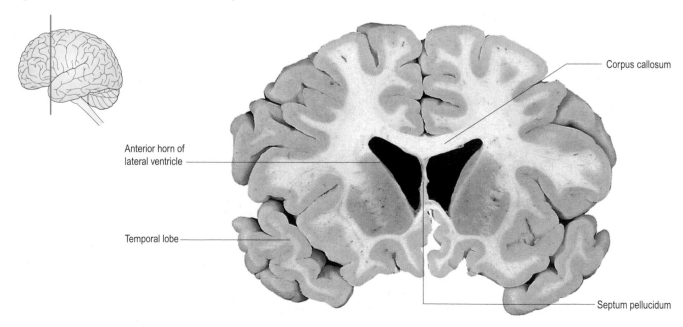

Corpus callosum

Anterior horn of lateral ventricle

Temporal lobe

Septum pellucidum

Fig. 13.5 **Coronal section of the cerebral hemisphere.**

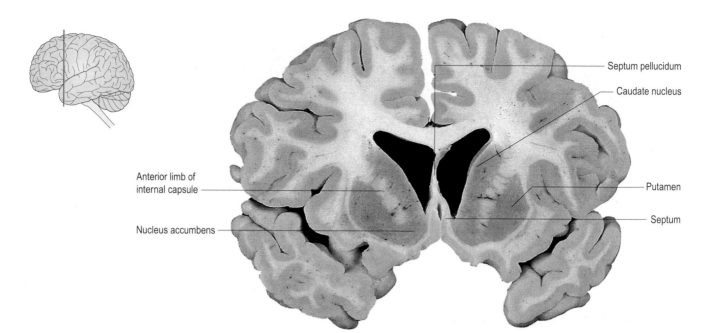

Septum pellucidum

Caudate nucleus

Anterior limb of internal capsule

Nucleus accumbens

Putamen

Septum

Fig. 13.6 **Coronal section of the cerebral hemisphere.**

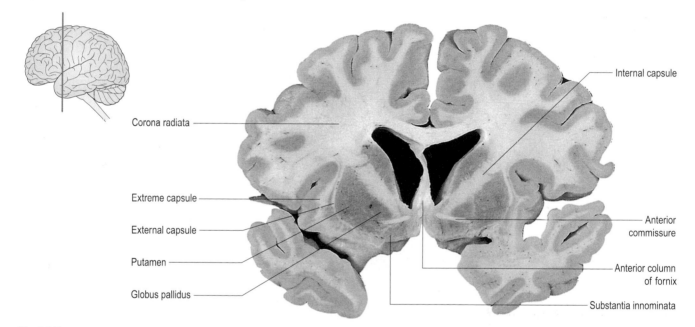

Corona radiata

Internal capsule

Extreme capsule

External capsule

Putamen

Globus pallidus

Anterior commissure

Anterior column of fornix

Substantia innominata

Fig. 13.7 **Coronal section of the cerebral hemisphere.**

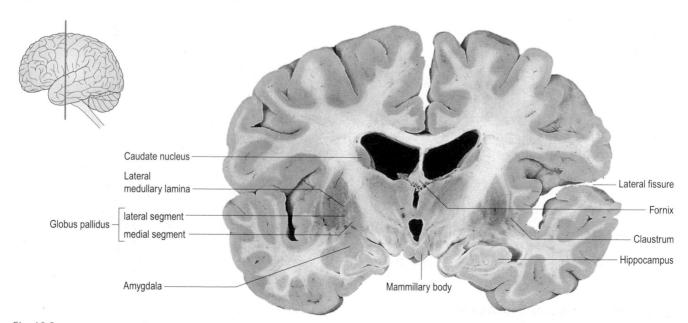

Caudate nucleus

Lateral medullary lamina

Globus pallidus — lateral segment / medial segment

Amygdala

Mammillary body

Lateral fissure

Fornix

Claustrum

Hippocampus

Fig. 13.8 **Coronal section of the cerebral hemisphere.**

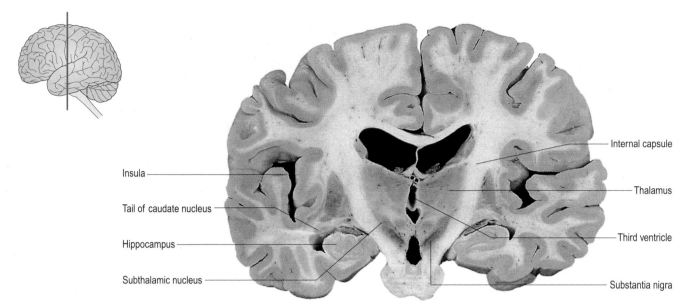

Internal capsule

Insula

Thalamus

Tail of caudate nucleus

Hippocampus

Third ventricle

Subthalamic nucleus

Substantia nigra

Fig. 13.9 **Coronal section of the cerebral hemisphere.**

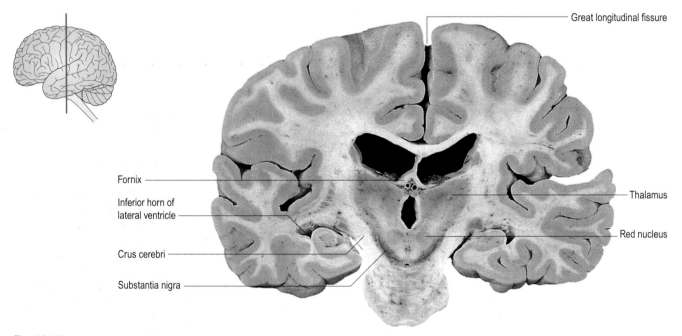

Great longitudinal fissure

Fornix

Inferior horn of lateral ventricle

Thalamus

Crus cerebri

Red nucleus

Substantia nigra

Fig. 13.10 **Coronal section of the cerebral hemisphere.**

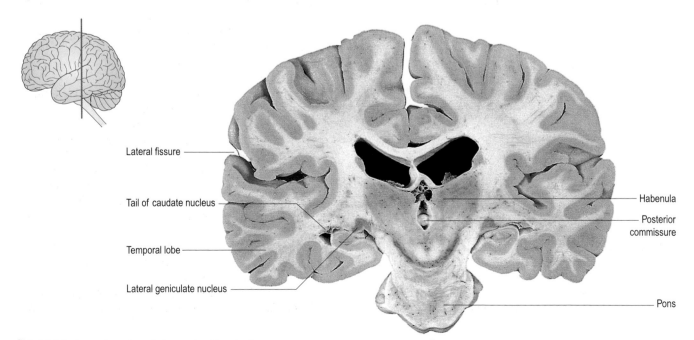

Lateral fissure

Tail of caudate nucleus

Habenula

Posterior commissure

Temporal lobe

Lateral geniculate nucleus

Pons

Fig. 13.11 **Coronal section of the cerebral hemisphere.**

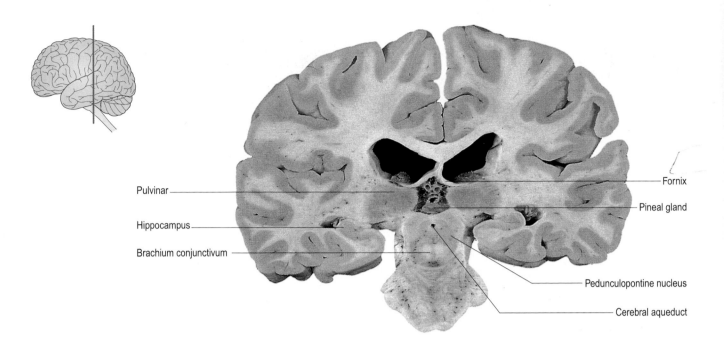

Pulvinar

Hippocampus

Brachium conjunctivum

Fornix

Pineal gland

Pedunculopontine nucleus

Cerebral aqueduct

Fig. 13.12 **Coronal section of the cerebral hemisphere.**

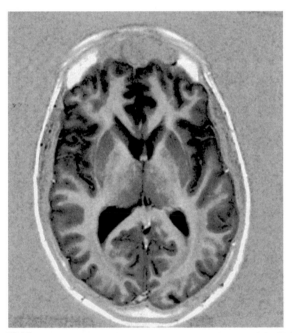

Fig. 13.13 **Horizontal (axial) magnetic resonance image of the living brain.** (Courtesy of Professor A Jackson).

Fig. 1.25). Between the internal capsule and the cortical surface, fibres radiate in and out to produce a fan-like arrangement, the **corona radiata**. Buried within the white matter lie a number of nuclear masses, most notably the caudate nucleus, putamen and globus pallidus, known collectively as the basal ganglia (Figs 13.3–13.15). Within the cerebral hemisphere lies the large C-shaped cavity of the lateral ventricle, which is considered with the rest of the ventricular system in Chapter 6.

The two cerebral hemispheres are separated by a deep cleft, the **great longitudinal fissure**, which accommodates the meningeal **falx cerebri**. In the depths of the fissure, the hemispheres are united by the **corpus callosum**, an enormous sheet of commissural nerve fibres which run

between corresponding areas of the two cortices (Figs 13.2–13.15; see also Figs 13.23 and 13.24).

Gyri, sulci and lobes of the cerebral hemisphere

Certain gyri and sulci on the surface of the hemisphere are consistently located in different individuals and form the basis of dividing the hemisphere into four lobes, namely the **frontal, parietal, temporal** and **occipital lobes**. Their principal topographical features and functional significance are described below. The most conspicuous and deepest cleft on the lateral surface of the hemisphere is the **lateral fissure** (Fig. 13.1). This separates the temporal lobe below, from the frontal and parietal lobes above. Within the depths of the lateral fissure lies a cortical area known as the **insula** (Figs 13.6–13.14). The parts of the frontal, parietal and temporal lobes that overlie the insula are called the **opercula**. Also on the lateral surface of the hemisphere, a single, uninterrupted sulcus can usually be identified, running continuously between the great longitudinal fissure and the lateral fissure. This is the **central sulcus**, which marks the boundary between the frontal and parietal lobes (Figs 13.1 and 13.16). The central sulcus extends for a short distance on to the medial surface of the hemisphere, within the great longitudinal fissure (Figs 13.2 and 13.16).

The frontal lobe constitutes the entire region in front of the central sulcus. Immediately in front of the sulcus, and running parallel to it, lies the **precentral gyrus**, which is the primary motor region of the cerebral cortex. In front of the precentral gyrus, the rest of the frontal lobe consists of a more variable pattern of convolutions, of which the **superior, middle** and **inferior frontal gyri** can usually be identified (Fig. 13.1).

Behind the central sulcus, and above the lateral fissure, lies the parietal lobe. Its most anterior part is the **postcentral gyrus**, which is the site of the primary somatosensory cortex. Behind the postcentral gyrus, on the lateral surface of the hemisphere, the **intraparietal sulcus** divides the rest of

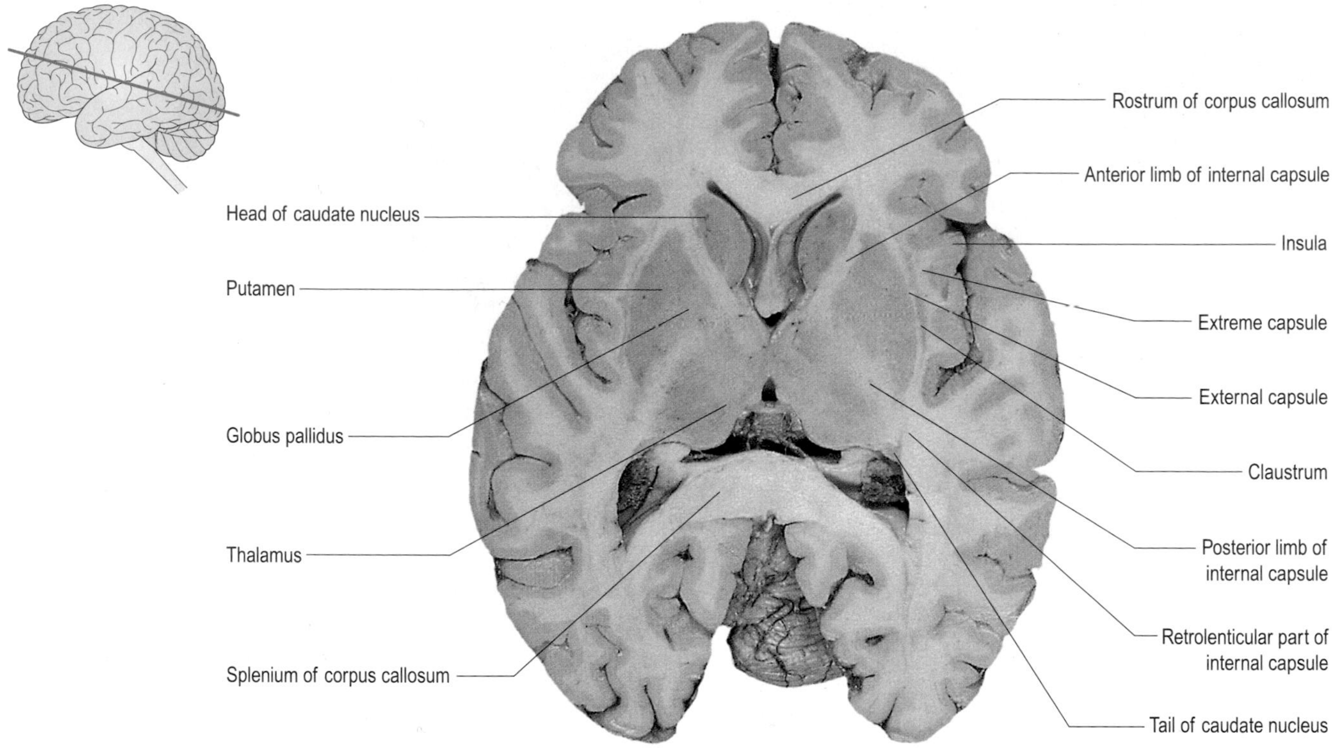

Head of caudate nucleus
Putamen
Globus pallidus
Thalamus
Splenium of corpus callosum
Rostrum of corpus callosum
Anterior limb of internal capsule
Insula
Extreme capsule
External capsule
Claustrum
Posterior limb of internal capsule
Retrolenticular part of internal capsule
Tail of caudate nucleus

Fig. 13.14 **Horizontal section of the brain.**

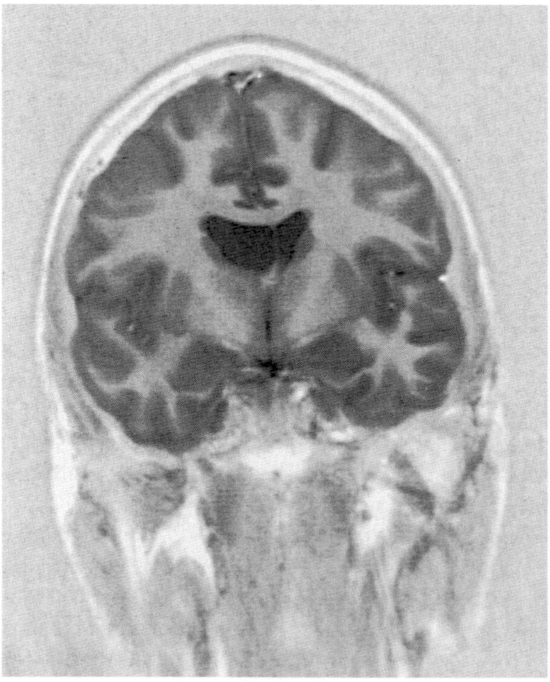

Fig. 13.15 **Coronal magnetic resonance image of the living brain.** (Courtesy of Professor A Jackson).

the parietal lobe into superior and inferior parietal lobules (Figs 13.1 and 13.16).

The boundary between the parietal lobe and the posteriorly located occipital lobe is not coincident with a single sulcus on the lateral surface of the hemisphere; however, it is clearly marked by the deep **parieto-occipital sulcus** on the medial surface (Figs 13.2 and 13.16). The occipital lobe does not bear any important landmarks on its lateral surface but, on the medial surface, the prominent **calcarine sulcus** indicates the location of the primary visual cortex (Figs 13.2 and 13.16).

The temporal lobe lies beneath the lateral fissure, merging posteriorly with the parietal and occipital lobes. On its lateral surface the temporal lobe is divided into three principal gyri that run roughly parallel to the lateral fissure: the superior, middle and inferior temporal gyri (Fig. 13.1). The superior temporal gyrus includes the primary auditory cortex. Most of this functional region is situated on the superior bank of the gyrus, within the lateral fissure, where the **transverse temporal gyri**, or **Heschl's convolutions**, provide a more precise localisation (Fig. 13.17).

On the medial surface of the hemisphere, certain portions of the frontal, parietal and temporal lobes also constitute components of the limbic system. Curving around the corpus callosum, and running parallel to it, lies the **cingulate gyrus** (Figs 13.2 and 13.16), separated from the rest of the hemisphere by the **cingulate sulcus**. The

Gyri, sulci and lobes of the cerebral hemisphere

- The cerebral hemisphere consists of:
  - the superficial cerebral cortex, convoluted to form gyri and sulci
  - underlying white matter, consisting of cortical afferent and efferent fibres
  - deep nuclear masses, the basal ganglia.
- The two cerebral hemispheres are separated by the great longitudinal fissure and joined by the corpus callosum.
- The hemisphere is divided into four lobes (frontal, parietal, temporal and occipital) on the basis of surface topography.
- Principal landmarks that indicate the divisions between lobes are the lateral fissure, central sulcus and parieto-occipital sulcus.

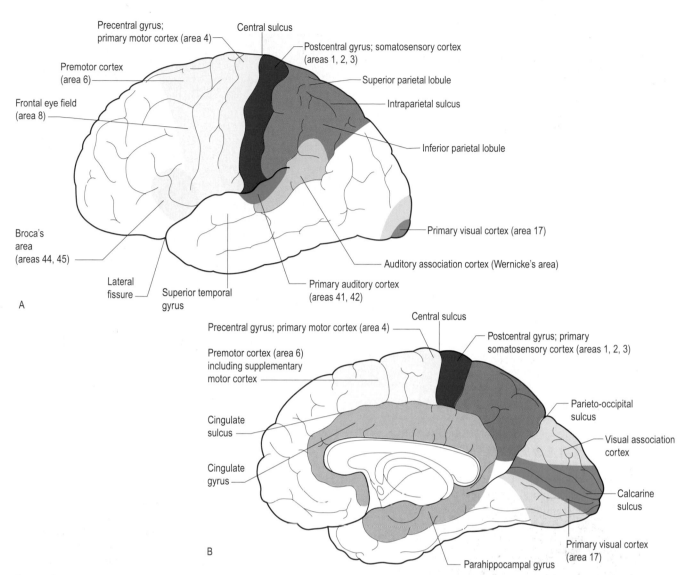

Fig. 13.16 **(A) Lateral aspect of the cerebral hemisphere showing major functional areas. (B) Median sagittal section of the cerebral hemisphere showing major functional areas.**

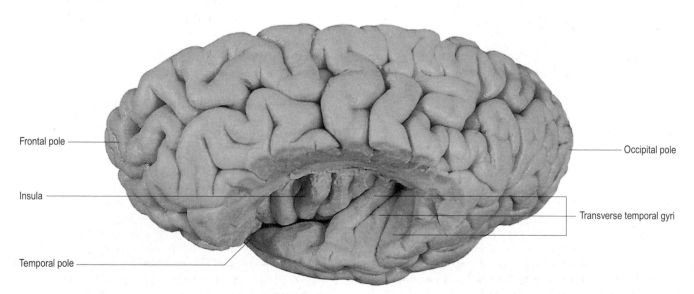

Fig. 13.17 **Superolateral aspect of the left cerebral hemisphere.** The frontal and parietal operculae have been removed to show the location of the transverse temporal gyri (Heschl's convolutions) and the insula.

cingulate gyrus passes posteriorly and inferiorly round the posterior portion, or splenium, of the corpus callosum to become continuous with the **parahippocampal gyrus** of the temporal lobe. Deep to the parahippocampal gyrus, within the temporal lobe, lies the **hippocampus** (Figs 13.8–13.12). This structure is formed by an in-curling of the inferomedial part of the temporal lobe. The cingulate gyrus, parahippocampal gyrus and hippocampus are sometimes referred to as the **limbic lobe** of the cerebral hemisphere.

Cerebral cortex

Histological structure

The cerebral cortex forms the outer surface of the cerebral hemisphere. It consists of a layer, several millimetres in thickness, of nerve cell bodies, dendritic arborisations and synaptic interconnections. In the early part of the 20th century, the Swedish anatomist Brodmann produced a numbered, cytoarchitectural map of the cerebral cortex based upon its regional histological characteristics. Although largely superseded by the elucidation of function, in some instances there is good correspondence between **Brodmann's areas** and functionally defined regions of the cortex. In such cases, Brodmann's numbers are retained in common use for descriptive purposes.

Long ago in evolutionary history, the cerebral cortex originally arose in relation to olfactory function. Phylogenetically old parts of the cortex (referred to as **archicortex** and **paleocortex**) such as the hippocampus and other parts of the temporal lobe retain throughout evolution an association with the olfactory system and have a primitive, three-layered cytoarchitecture. These regions have important functions in the emotional aspects of behaviour and in memory. Together with other parts of the cortex and certain subcortical nuclei they constitute the limbic system (Chapter 16). However, most of the cerebral cortex is a more recent acquisition in phylogenetic terms and is referred to as the **neocortex**. Although its detailed cytological structure varies from region to region, it is generally recognised as consisting of six layers (Fig. 13.18).

- **Layer I**, the most superficial layer, contains few nerve cell bodies but many dendritic and axonal processes in synaptic interaction.
- **Layer II** contains many small neurones, which establish intracortical connections.
- **Layer III** contains medium-sized neurones giving rise to association and commissural fibres.
- **Layer IV** is the site of termination of afferent fibres from the specific thalamic nuclei.
- **Layer V** is the origin of projection fibres to extracortical targets, such as basal ganglia, thalamus, brain stem and spinal cord. In the primary motor cortex of the frontal lobe, this layer contains the giant Betz cells, which project fibres into the pyramidal tract.
- **Layer VI** also contains association and projection neurones.

Functional organisation

The cerebral cortex is necessary for conscious awareness and thought, memory and intellect. It is the region to which all sensory modalities ultimately ascend (mostly via the thalamus) and where they are consciously perceived and

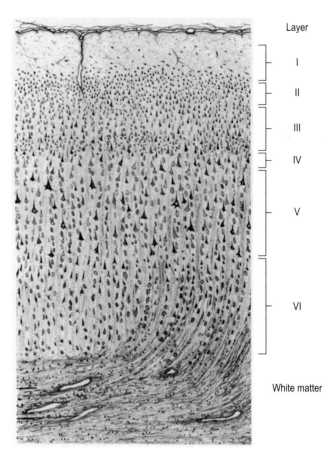

Fig. 13.18 **The histological structure of the cerebral cortex.** (From Mitchell and Patterson, *Basic Anatomy*, 1954, courtesy of Churchill Livingstone).

Focal cerebral lesions

Focal cerebral lesions, e.g. a stroke or tumour, produce three kinds of symptom:

- **Partial epileptic seizures.** The repetitive discharges of groups of neurones in the cerebral cortex produce paroxysmal attacks lasting for brief periods and reflecting the functional properties of the neurones concerned. The patient experiences sudden attacks of abnormal movements or sensations (**simple partial seizures**) or brief alterations in perception, mood and behaviour (**complex partial seizures**). Partial seizures may trigger **generalised (tonic–clonic) seizures**.
- **Sensory/motor deficits.** There is a loss of sensation or movement, detectable on clinical neurological examination.
- **Psychological deficits.** There are breakdowns in psychological processes such as language, perception and memory, demonstrable on psychological evaluation.

If the focal lesion is space-occupying, the syndrome of **raised intracranial pressure** results (see p. 47).

A **unilateral cerebral hemisphere lesion** causes mental impairment (e.g. aphasia), a contralateral spastic hemiparesis, hyperreflexia and an extensor plantar response (upper motor neurone lesion), and contralateral hemisensory loss (Fig. 13.19; see also Fig. 1.43). A vascular insult to the internal capsule, such as an infarction or haemorrhage, leads to the rapid development of this syndrome, known as **stroke**.

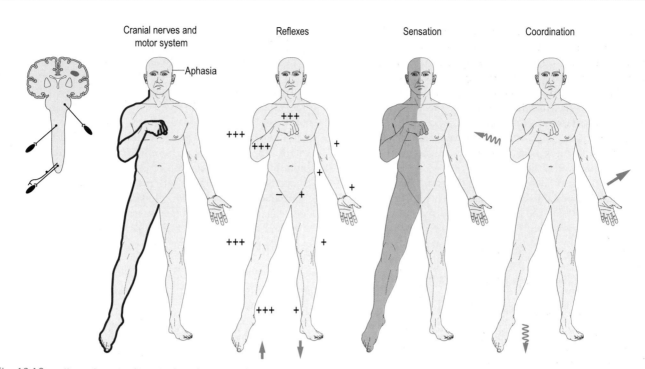

Fig. 13.19 **Unilateral cerebral hemisphere lesion.** For key see Figure 1.43.

interpreted in the light of previous experience. The cerebral cortex is the highest level at which the motor system is represented. It is here that actions are conceived and initiated.

- The posterior part of the cerebrum receives sensory information from the outside world in the primary sensory areas of the parietal lobe (somatosensory), occipital lobe (vision) and temporal lobe (hearing).
- In adjacent cortical zones, the information is elaborated to permit identification of objects by touch, sight and hearing in a modality-specific act of perception. Areas of cortex at the junction of the three cerebral lobes, known as association cortex, are critical for the multimodal and spatial recognition of the environment.
- The medial portions of the cerebral hemisphere (limbic system) enable the storage and retrieval of information processed in the posterior hemispheric regions.
- The anterior part of the cerebrum (frontal lobe) is concerned with the organisation of movement (primary motor area; premotor and supplementary motor areas) and the strategic guidance of complex motor behaviour over time (prefrontal area).
- In the majority of individuals, areas of association cortex in frontal, parietal and temporal lobes of the left hemisphere are responsible for the comprehension and expression of language. The left hemisphere is, therefore, said to be **dominant** for language.

Frontal lobe

The frontal lobe lies anterior to the central sulcus. Immediately anterior to the central sulcus, and running parallel to it, is the precentral gyrus. Functionally, this is known as the **primary motor cortex** (Figs 13.1, 13.2 and 13.16). It corresponds to Brodmann's area 4. Within the cortex of the precentral gyrus, the contralateral half of the body is represented in a precise somatotopic fashion, often pictorially depicted as a 'motor homunculus' (Fig. 13.20). The representation of the body is inverted, with the head area located in the most inferior part of the precentral gyrus, just

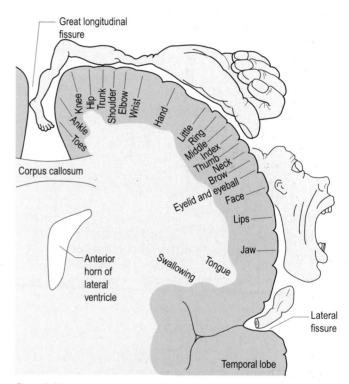

Fig. 13.20 **Motor homunculus illustrating somatotopic organisation of the primary motor cortex.**

above the lateral fissure. Progressing superiorly, successive areas of cortex represent the digits, hand, arm, shoulder and trunk. The lower limb is represented on the medial surface of the hemisphere, above the corpus callosum. The area of cortex devoted to a particular body part is proportional, not to its size, but to the degree of precision with which movements can be executed. Therefore, the larynx, tongue, face and digits of the hand are represented by relatively large regions.

Stimulation of the primary motor cortex elicits contraction of discrete muscle groups on the opposite side of the body.

The function of this region is the control of voluntary, skilled movements, sometimes referred to as fractionated movements; 30% of corticospinal (pyramidal tract) and corticobulbar fibres arise from neurones of the primary motor cortex, about 3% originating from giant pyramidal (Betz) cells. The principal subcortical afferents to the primary motor cortex originate from the ventral lateral nucleus of the thalamus (Fig. 12.6), which in turn receives input mainly from the dentate nucleus of the cerebellum and from the globus pallidus of the basal ganglia.

The region immediately anterior to the primary motor cortex is known as the **premotor cortex** (Brodmann's area 6) (Fig. 13.16). On the lateral surface of the hemisphere, this includes the posterior portions of the superior, middle and inferior frontal gyri. On the medial surface of the hemisphere, the premotor cortex includes a region referred to as the **supplementary motor cortex**. Here, like the primary motor cortex, there is somatotopic representation of the body although, unlike the primary motor cortex, representation appears to be bilateral in both hemispheres.

Stimulation of premotor cortical areas induces movements that are less focused than those elicited from the primary motor cortex and that involve groups of functionally related muscles. Movements evoked from the supplementary motor cortex tend to be postural in nature, involving axial and proximal musculature. Premotor cortical areas are thought to function in the programming of, and preparation for, movement and in the control of posture. The premotor cortex exerts its actions partly via the primary motor cortex, with which it is connected by short association fibres, and partly via corticospinal and corticobulbar fibres. About 30% of the latter originate in the premotor cortex although, unlike the primary motor cortex, giant Betz cells are absent from premotor areas. The principal subcortical input to premotor cortical regions, including the supplementary motor cortex, is the ventral anterior nucleus of the thalamus. This, in turn, receives fibres from the globus pallidus and substantia nigra.

Immediately in front of the premotor cortex, on the lateral surface of the hemisphere, are located two other important regions. In the middle frontal gyrus lies the **frontal eye field** (Brodmann's area 8). This region controls voluntary conjugate deviation of the eyes, as occur when scanning the visual field. Unilateral damage to this area causes conjugate

deviation of the eyes towards the side of the lesion. In the inferior frontal gyrus of the dominant hemisphere (usually the left) lies the motor speech area, also known as **Broca's area** (Brodmann's areas 44 and 45). Broca's area has important interconnections with parts of the ipsilateral temporal, parietal and occipital lobes that are involved in language function.

The extensive regions of the cortex of the frontal lobe that lie anterior to premotor areas are referred to as **prefrontal cortex**. The prefrontal cortex has rich connections with parietal, temporal and occipital cortex through long association fibres running in the subcortical white matter. Subcortical afferents arise mainly in the mediodorsal and anterior nuclei of the thalamus. The prefrontal cortex has cognitive functions of a high order. These include intellectual, judgemental and predictive faculties and the planning of behaviour.

Parietal lobe

The parietal lobe lies behind the frontal lobe and is bounded posteriorly and inferiorly by the occipital and temporal lobes, respectively. The most anterior part of the parietal lobe is the postcentral gyrus, running parallel to the central

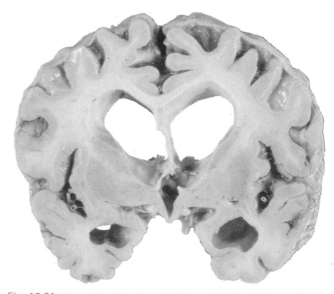

Fig. 13.21 **Coronal section through the cerebral hemisphere of a dying patient with Alzheimer's disease.** Note the enlarged lateral ventricles and atrophic cortical gyri. (Courtesy of Professor D Mann).

sulcus (Figs 13.1, 13.2 and 13.16). Functionally, this region is the **primary somatosensory cortex** (Brodmann's areas 1, 2 and 3). It is here that thalamocortical neurones terminate; these constitute the third and final relay in the chain from peripheral receptors for general sensation to a conscious level. The thalamic origin of these neurones is the ventral posterior nucleus, which in turn receives fibres of the medial lemniscus (fine touch and proprioception), spinal lemniscus (coarse touch and pressure), spinothalamic tracts (pain and temperature) and trigeminothalamic tracts (general sensation from the head). Within the somatosensory cortex, the contralateral half of the body is represented in an inverted, somatotopic pattern that resembles that in the primary motor cortex of the frontal lobe (Fig. 13.22).

Once again, the area of cortex devoted to a particular body part is disproportionate to the size of the latter; in the case of the sensory cortex it reflects rather the richness of sensory innervation. Therefore, the pharynx, tongue, face, lips and the palmar surface of the hands and digits are particularly well represented. Adjacent to the mouth area is a region where taste is perceived.

The surface of the parietal lobe posterior to the primary somatosensory cortex constitutes the parietal **association cortex**. The superior parietal lobule is responsible for the interpretation of general sensory information and for conscious awareness of the contralateral half of the body. Lesions here impair the interpretation and understanding of sensory input and may cause neglect of the opposite side of the body. The inferior parietal lobule interfaces between somatosensory cortex and the visual and auditory association cortices of the occipital and temporal lobes, respectively, and in the dominant hemisphere it contributes to language functions.

Temporal lobe

The lateral surface of the temporal lobe is divided into superior, middle and inferior temporal gyri, which run parallel

Parietal lobe lesions
Left parietal lobe lesions cause:

- partial seizures – paroxysmal attacks of abnormal sensations, spreading down the contralateral side of the body (sensory seizures)
- sensory/motor deficit – a contralateral hemisensory loss and inferior visual field loss
- Psychological deficit – an inability to name objects (**anomia**) and a loss of literacy, with inability to read (**alexia**), to write (**agraphia**) and to calculate (**acalculia**).

Right parietal lobe lesions cause:

- partial seizures – paroxysmal attacks of sensory disturbance affecting the contralateral side of the body (simple sensory seizures)
- sensory/motor deficit – contralateral hemisensory loss and an inferior visual field loss
- psychological deficit – an inability to copy and construct designs because of spatial disorientation (**constructional apraxia**).

to the lateral fissure. Within the superior temporal gyrus is located the **primary auditory cortex** (Brodmann's areas 41 and 42). More exactly, most of this functional zone lies in the superior bank of the gyrus, normally hidden within the lateral fissure. Its precise location is marked by the small transverse temporal gyri, or Heschl's convolutions (Fig. 13.17).

The primary auditory cortex is responsible for the conscious perception of sound and within it there is so-called 'tonotopical' representation of the cochlear duct. The primary auditory cortex receives input from the medial geniculate nucleus of the thalamus. The ascending acoustic projection undergoes partial decussation in the brain stem on its way to the medial geniculate nucleus (Chapter 10). At the cortical level, therefore, the organs of hearing are bilaterally represented so that unilateral lesions of the primary auditory cortex cause partial deafness in both ears. Auditory information is further processed and interpreted in the **auditory association cortex**, which lies surrounding and immediately posterior to the primary auditory cortex. In the dominant hemisphere, this region is also known as **Wernicke's area**. It is crucial for understanding of the spoken word and has important connections with other language areas of the brain.

The location of the cortical representation of the vestibular system is uncertain. There is evidence that it lies in the superior temporal gyrus anterior to the primary auditory cortex, or in the inferior parietal lobule.

The inferomedial part of the temporal lobe is curled inwards to form the **hippocampus**. This structure lies in the floor of the inferior horn of the lateral ventricle, deep to the parahippocampal gyrus (Figs 13.8–13.12, 13.16, see also Chapter 16). As part of the limbic system, the principal functions of the hippocampus are in relation to memory and the emotional aspects of behaviour. Close to the anterior end of the hippocampus and the temporal pole lies a mass of subcortical grey matter, the **amygdala**, which is also part of the limbic system. The amygdala and adjacent parts of the inferomedial temporal cortex receive fibres from the

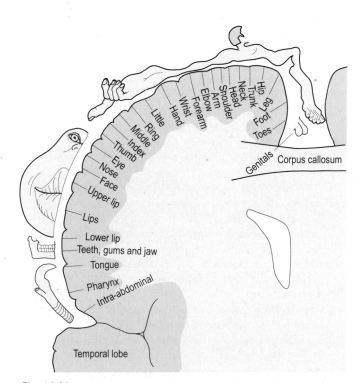

Fig. 13.22 **Sensory homunculus illustrating somatotopic organisation of the primary somatosensory cortex.**

Left temporal lobe lesions
Left temporal lobe lesions cause:

- Partial seizures – paroxysmal attacks of unresponsiveness (**absences**), purposeless behaviour (**automatism**), olfactory and complex visual and auditory hallucinations, and disturbances of mood and memory (**déjà vu**). These attacks are referred to as complex partial seizures.
- Sensory/motor deficit – a contralateral superior visual field loss.
- Psychological deficit – speech that is fluent and rapid but contains word errors (paraphasia) and is incomprehensible. There is profound word-finding difficulty, impaired repetition of words, and profound loss of comprehension. This is known as **Wernicke's aphasia**.

olfactory tract and are responsible for the conscious appreciation of the sense of smell. These connections receive further consideration in Chapter 16.

Occipital lobe
The occipital lobe lies behind the parietal and temporal lobes. On the medial surface of the hemisphere, the boundary with the parietal lobe is marked by the deep parieto-occipital sulcus. Also on the medial surface, the calcarine sulcus marks the location of the **primary visual cortex** (Brodmann's area 17) (Fig. 13.16), which is responsible for visual perception. It occupies the gyri immediately above and below the calcarine sulcus, much of it being hidden in the depths of the sulci. This region receives fibres from the lateral geniculate nucleus of the thalamus by way of the optic radiation of the internal capsule. Each lateral half of the visual field is represented in the primary visual cortex of the contralateral hemisphere. The upper half of the visual field is represented below the calcarine sulcus, and the lower half is represented above the sulcus. The rest of the occipital lobe constitutes the **visual association cortex**. This region is concerned with the interpretation of visual images. Lesions of the primary visual cortex cause blindness in the corresponding part of the visual field, while damage to the visual association cortex causes deficits in visual interpretation and recognition.

Occipital lobe lesions
Occipital lobe lesions cause:

- partial seizures – paroxysmal visual hallucinations of a simple, unformed nature, such as lights and colours (simple partial seizures).
- sensory/motor deficit – a contralateral visual field loss (**contralateral homonymous hemianopia**).

Bilateral occipital lobe lesions lead to **cortical blindness**, of which the patient is unaware (**Anton's syndrome**). Bilateral occipito-parietal lesions can spare elementary vision but prevent the recognition and depiction of objects (**apperceptive visual agnosia**).

Language areas of the cerebral hemisphere
Certain higher cognitive functions are dealt with primarily, or even exclusively, by one of the cerebral hemispheres, which is then referred to as dominant for that function. In the great majority of people the left hemisphere is dominant for language and mathematical ability. The right hemisphere excels at spatial perception and musical proficiency. Cerebral dominance becomes established during the first few years after birth. During this formative period, both hemispheres exhibit linguistic ability and if one hemisphere sustains damage it may be compensated for by the plasticity of the developing brain and the child learns to speak normally. Later in life, this flexibility becomes greatly diminished and damage to the dominant hemisphere often causes loss of speech in addition to the other deficits produced by hemispheric lesions.

The language areas of the brain are organised around the lateral fissure of the cerebral hemisphere. In the frontal lobe, Broca's area occupies the posterior part of the inferior frontal gyrus, adjacent to the motor cortical area for the head and neck. This region is concerned with expressive aspects of language (articulation). In the temporal lobe, the auditory association cortex, or Wernicke's area, is responsible for comprehension of the spoken word.

Nearby regions of the temporal lobe and parietal lobe, most notably the angular gyrus and supramarginal gyrus of the inferior parietal lobule, provide a functional interface between auditory and visual association areas important in naming, reading, writing and calculation.

The cerebral cortex

- The precentral gyrus is the primary motor region of the cerebral cortex and is located within the frontal lobe, immediately in front of the central sulcus. Anterior to this lie the premotor and supplementary motor cortices and, in the left hemisphere, Broca's (motor speech) area. The prefrontal cortex is concerned with complex cognitive functions.
- The postcentral gyrus is the primary somatosensory region of the cerebral cortex and lies within the parietal lobe, immediately posterior to the central sulcus. It receives afferents from the ventral posterior nucleus of the thalamus, which is the site of termination of the spinothalamic tracts, trigeminothalamic tract and the medial lemniscus. Behind this region lies the sensory association cortex, which is responsible for the interpretation of general sensory information.
- The temporal lobe lies beneath the lateral fissure. On the superior surface of the superior temporal gyrus, the transverse temporal gyri (Heschl's convolutions) mark the location of the primary auditory cortex, which receives input from the medial geniculate nucleus of the thalamus. Adjacent lies the auditory association cortex, which is responsible for the interpretation of auditory information and which, in the left hemisphere, constitutes Wernicke's area.
- The occipital lobe makes up the posterior part of the hemisphere. On the medial surface, the calcarine sulcus indicates the location of the primary visual cortex, which receives afferents from the lateral geniculate nucleus of the thalamus. The rest of the occipital lobe is the visual association cortex, which is responsible for the interpretation of visual information.

White matter of the cerebral hemisphere

Beneath the cortical surface lies an enormous mass of nerve fibres, all of which have their origin or termination, or sometimes both, within the cortex. The fibres are classified into three types, depending upon their origin and destination:

- **association fibres**, which interconnect cortical sites lying within one cerebral hemisphere.
- **commissural fibres**, which run from one cerebral hemisphere to the other, connecting functionally related structures.
- **projection fibres**, which pass between the cerebral cortex and subcortical structures such as the thalamus, striatum, brain stem and spinal cord.

Association fibres

Some association fibres (Figs 13.23 and 13.24) are short and link nearby areas of cortex by arching beneath adjacent cerebral sulci (U fibres). Other association fibres are longer and travel through the white matter to link distant areas of cerebral cortex. The primary sensory areas in the parietal, temporal and occipital lobes are linked by long association fibres to the association areas of the cerebral cortex. These, in turn, are connected to each other.

The large **superior longitudinal fasciculus** interconnects the frontal and occipital lobes. A subsidiary of this bundle, known as the **arcuate fasciculus**, links gyri in the frontal and temporal lobes that are important for language function.

The **inferior longitudinal fasciculus** runs from the occipital to the temporal poles and contributes to the function of visual recognition.

The **uncinate fasciculus** connects the anterior and inferior parts of the frontal lobe with the temporal gyri, which are important structures in the regulation of behaviour. The **cingulum** lies within the cingulate gyrus and courses around the corpus callosum, connecting the frontal and parietal lobes with the parahippocampal and adjacent temporal gyri.

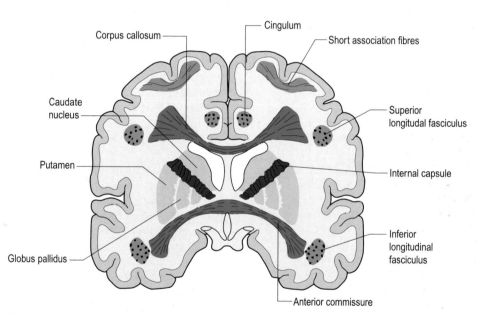

Fig. 13.23 **Coronal section of the cerebral hemisphere.** The diagram shows the location of the principal association, commissural and projection fibres.

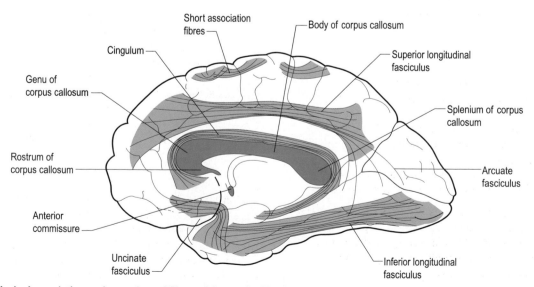

Fig. 13.24 **Principal association and commissural fibres of the cerebral hemisphere projected on to the medial surface.**

Commissural fibres

The major interhemispheric commissural fibres are the corpus callosum, the anterior commissure and the hippocampal commissure (or commissure of the fornix) (Figs 13.23–13.26).

The **corpus callosum** spans the two cerebral hemispheres and connects corresponding regions of neocortex for all but the temporal fields (these have their own connection, the anterior commissure). The major parts of the corpus callosum, from rostral to caudal, are named the rostrum, genu, body and splenium. The corpus callosum is shorter rostrocaudally than is the hemisphere; as a result, callosal fibres linking the frontal or occipital poles curve forwards or backwards as the anterior and posterior forceps, respectively. The **splenium** interconnects the occipital cortices and, therefore, contributes to visual functions.

The **anterior commissure** runs transversely in front of the anterior column of the fornix and interconnects the inferior and middle temporal gyri and the olfactory regions on the two sides.

The **hippocampal commissure** consists of transverse fibres linking the posterior columns of the fornix on each side.

Projection fibres

Projection fibres (Fig. 13.23) consist of afferent fibres conveying impulses to the cortex and efferent fibres

conducting impulses away from it. The fibres projecting to and from the cerebral cortex are distributed radially as the corona radiata and then converge downwards towards the brain stem. The fibres become concentrated in a narrow area, called the **internal capsule**, between the thalamus and caudate nucleus medially, and the lentiform nucleus laterally. The internal capsule is angulated to form an anterior limb, genu, posterior limb and retrolenticular part (Fig. 13.26; Fig. 1.25).

The **anterior limb** contains connections between the mediodorsal nucleus of the thalamus and the prefrontal cortex, and also frontopontine fibres that project to the pontine nuclei in the basal portion of the pons.

The **posterior limb** contains corticobulbar and corticospinal motor fibres. Also within the posterior limb are thalamocortical projections passing from the ventral posterior nucleus to the primary somatosensory cortex, and from the ventral anterior and ventral lateral nuclei to motor regions of the frontal lobe.

Behind the posterior limb is a region referred to as the **retrolenticular** part of the internal capsule. This consists of fibres arising from the medial and lateral geniculate nuclei of

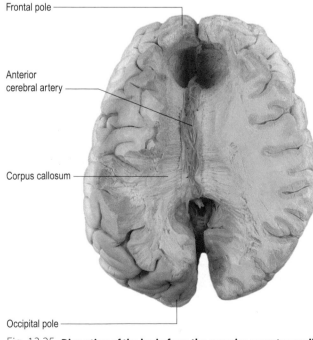

Frontal pole

Anterior cerebral artery

Corpus callosum

Occipital pole

Fig. 13.25 **Dissection of the brain from the superior aspect revealing the corpus callosum.**

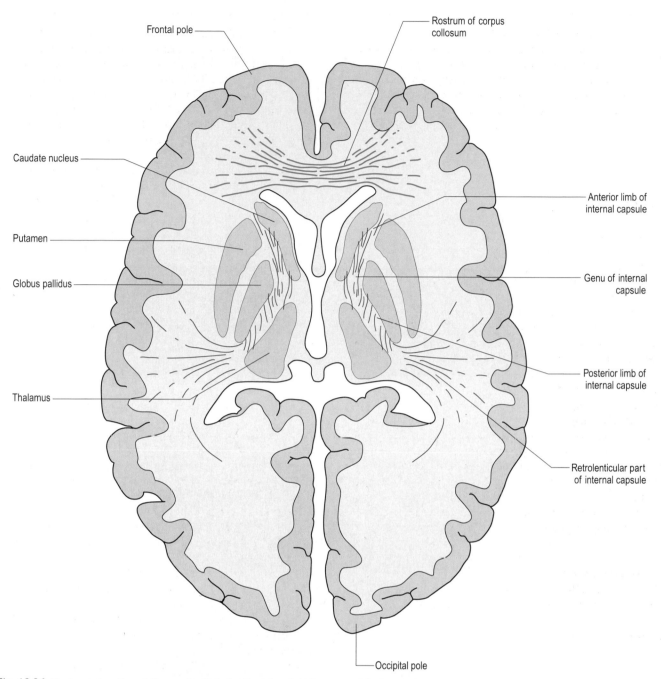

Fig. 13.26 **Horizontal section of the cerebral hemisphere showing the parts of the internal capsule.**

the thalamus that pass to the auditory and visual cortices as the auditory and visual radiations, respectively. Visual thalamocortical fibres (also known as geniculocalcarine fibres) pass round the lateral ventricle and follow one of two courses to the visual cortex (Fig. 15.6). Those which represent the lower half of the visual field project to the upper part of the visual cortex (above the calcarine sulcus). They may be interrupted in their course by lesions of the parietal lobe. Fibres that represent the upper half of the visual field loop forwards over the inferior horn of the lateral ventricle (Meyer's loop) and may be damaged by lesions of the temporal lobe.

Chapter 14
Corpus striatum

Within the cerebral hemisphere lie a number of nuclear masses, collectively referred to as the **basal ganglia** (Figs 14.1 and 14.2; see also 13.3–13.9 and 13.14). The major components are the **caudate nucleus**, **putamen** and **globus pallidus**. The **amygdala**, which is located within the temporal lobe, has a similar embryological derivation but is functionally quite different. It is part of the limbic system and is considered in Chapter 16.

The caudate nucleus, putamen and globus pallidus are anatomically and functionally related closely to each other and are principally involved in the control of posture and movement. They are sometimes referred to anatomically as the **corpus striatum** but, clinically, abnormalities of movement resulting from their dysfunction are commonly called basal ganglia disorders. The corpus striatum has important connections with other regions of the brain, particularly the cerebral cortex, the thalamus and subthalamic nucleus of the diencephalon, and the substantia nigra of the midbrain.

For gross anatomical purposes, the putamen and globus pallidus are sometimes together called the **lentiform** (or **lenticular) nucleus**. This is because they lie close together, forming an apparently single structure. The name means 'lentil-shaped', but a closer analogy would be a Brazil nut or the segment of an orange. The lentiform nucleus is three-sided, having a convex lateral surface and two other surfaces that converge to a medial apex which lies against the genu of the internal capsule. The term lentiform or lenticular is rather archaic and of limited usefulness, although it is still retained in certain anatomical names (such as the retrolenticular part of the internal capsule).

On phylogenetic, connectional and functional grounds, the putamen is more closely allied to the caudate nucleus than

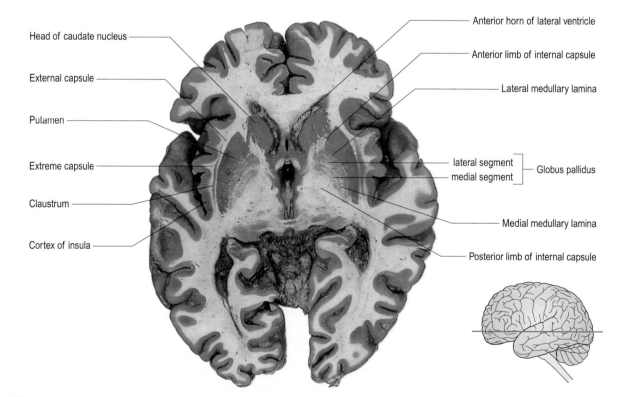

Fig. 14.1 **Horizontal section of the brain showing the relationships of the corpus striatum.** Mulligan's stain has been used to increase the contrast between cell-rich areas (blue) and white matter.

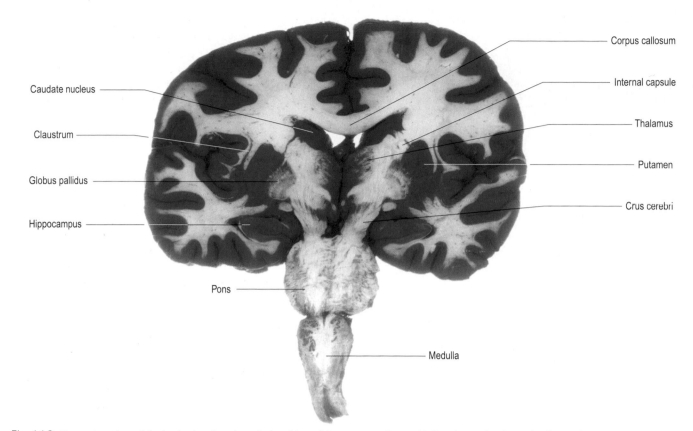

Fig. 14.2 **Coronal section of the brain showing the relationships of the corpus striatum.** Mulligan's stain (see legend to Fig. 14.1).

to the globus pallidus. The globus pallidus is, in phylogenetic terms, the oldest part of the corpus striatum and is sometimes referred to as the **paleostriatum**. The abbreviation **pallidum** is more commonly used, particularly in composite terms for afferent and efferent connections, such as subthalamopallidal or pallidothalamic.

The caudate nucleus and putamen constitute the phylogenetically more recent **neostriatum** and are best regarded as a single entity. The two parts are almost (but not entirely) separated by the internal capsule but their gross anatomical separation is not as significant as their neuronal

and functional similarities. They are commonly referred to simply as the **striatum**.

These rather confusing relationships are summarised in Figure 14.3.

Topographical anatomy of the corpus striatum

Striatum

The striatum (neostriatum) consists of the caudate nucleus and the putamen. Their combined three-dimensional shape is reminiscent of a tadpole, when viewed laterally (Fig. 14.4).

Putamen

The putamen lies lateral to the internal capsule and globus pallidus (Figs 14.1 and 14.2; see also Figs 13.7, 13.8 and 13.14). It is separated from the globus pallidus by a thin lamina of nerve fibres, the lateral medullary lamina. Lateral to the putamen lies more white matter, sandwiched within which lies a thin sheet of grey matter, known as the claustrum. This separates the white matter into two layers, the external capsule and the extreme capsule (Fig. 14.1). Lateral to the extreme capsule lies the cortex of the insula, deep within the lateral fissure of the hemisphere.

Caudate nucleus

The caudate nucleus consists of a large head and a tapering, curved tail. The head of the caudate is almost completely separated from the putamen by the internal capsule. At its rostral extremity, however, it is continuous with the putamen through and beneath the anterior limb of the internal capsule (Fig. 14.4 and Figs 13.4–13.6). At this level, the most ventral portion of the striatum is known as the

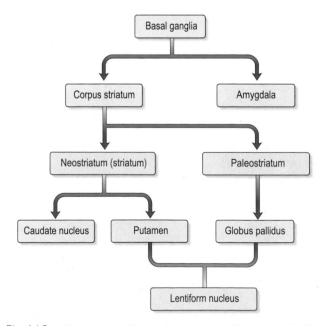

Fig. 14.3 **Relationships of the nuclear masses within the cerebral hemisphere.**

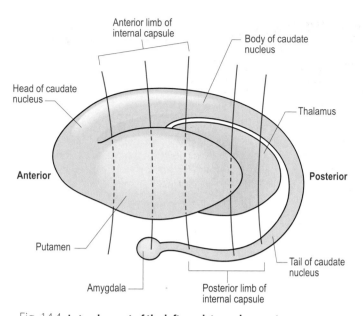

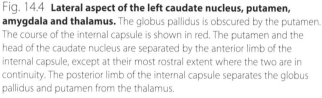

Fig. 14.4 **Lateral aspect of the left caudate nucleus, putamen, amygdala and thalamus.** The globus pallidus is obscured by the putamen. The course of the internal capsule is shown in red. The putamen and the head of the caudate nucleus are separated by the anterior limb of the internal capsule, except at their most rostral extent where the two are in continuity. The posterior limb of the internal capsule separates the globus pallidus and putamen from the thalamus.

nucleus accumbens, which has connections with the limbic system. The head of the caudate nucleus forms a prominent bulge in the lateral wall of the anterior horn of the lateral ventricle (Fig. 14.1 and Figs 13.3–13.7). The tail of the caudate passes posteriorly, gradually tapering as it does so and, following the curvature of the ventricle, descends into the temporal lobe where it lies in the roof of the inferior horn (Fig. 14.4 and Figs 13.9–13.12).

Globus pallidus

The globus pallidus lies medial to the putamen, separated from it by the lateral medullary lamina. Its medial apex nestles into the lateral concavity of the internal capsule

---

Topographical anatomy of the corpus striatum

- The corpus striatum includes the caudate nucleus, putamen and globus pallidus.
- These structures are primarily concerned with the control of posture and movement.
- Topographically, the putamen and globus pallidus constitute the lentiform nucleus.
- Functionally, the caudate nucleus and putamen form a single entity, the neostriatum (striatum), while the globus pallidus forms the paleostriatum.
- The caudate nucleus lies in the wall of the lateral ventricle.
- The largest part, or head, of the caudate lies medial to the internal capsule and forms a prominent bulge in the lateral wall of the anterior horn of the ventricle.
- The curved, tapering tail of the caudate nucleus follows the curvature of the lateral ventricle into the temporal lobe.
- The putamen and globus pallidus lie lateral to the internal capsule, deep to the cortex of the insula.

(Fig. 14.1). The globus pallidus consists of two divisions, referred to as the lateral (or external) and the medial (or internal) segments. These are separated by a thin sheet of fibres, the medial medullary lamina (Fig. 14.1). The smaller medial segment shares many similarities, in terms of cytology and connections, with the pars reticulata of the substantia nigra in the midbrain. Although the two are separated by the internal capsule, they are best regarded as a single entity, in the functional sense.

Substantia innominata

The term substantia innominata refers to the basal part of the rostral forebrain that lies beneath the corpus striatum (see Fig. 14.7). This complex region contains several groups of neurones, one of them being the **nucleus basalis** (of Meynert), that project widely to the cerebral cortex and utilise acetylcholine as their neurotransmitter. These neurones undergo degeneration in Alzheimer's disease.

Functional anatomy of the corpus striatum

Connections of the striatum

The caudate nucleus and putamen, together commonly referred to as the striatum, are best considered as a single entity since they share common neuronal organisation, neurotransmitter systems and connections (Fig. 14.5). They are often regarded as the 'input' portions of the corpus striatum, since the majority of afferents from other parts of the brain end here rather than in the globus pallidus.

Striatal afferents

Afferents to the striatum come from three principal sources: the cerebral cortex, the thalamus and the substantia nigra.

Corticostriatal fibres originate from widespread regions of the cerebral cortex, predominantly, but not exclusively, of the ipsilateral side. Fibres from the frontal and parietal lobes predominate. Motor regions of the frontal lobe project mainly to the putamen, where the body is represented in an inverted, somatotopic fashion. More anterior regions of the frontal lobe, and other association cortices, project mainly to the caudate nucleus. For these reasons, the putamen is considered to be the most overtly motor part of the striatum, the caudate nucleus having more associative functions. Corticostriatal fibres are excitatory to striatal neurones and use glutamic acid as their transmitter.

The **thalamostriatal projection** comes from the intralaminar nuclei (centromedian and parafascicular nuclei) of the ipsilateral thalamus.

The **nigrostriatal projection** originates from the **pars compacta** of the ipsilateral **substantia nigra** of the midbrain tegmentum. The transmitter used by this pathway is the monoamine dopamine, which has both excitatory and inhibitory effects upon striatal neurones. The neurones of the pars compacta contain the dark pigment neuromelanin (Fig. 14.6), which is produced as a by-product of dopamine synthesis. The most rostral and ventral portion of the striatum, the nucleus accumbens, receives its dopaminergic input from the ventral tegmental area, which lies medial to the substantia nigra. This projection is known as the mesostriatal pathway. Other afferents to the striatum include a projection from the brain stem **raphe nuclei**, utilising serotonin as its transmitter.

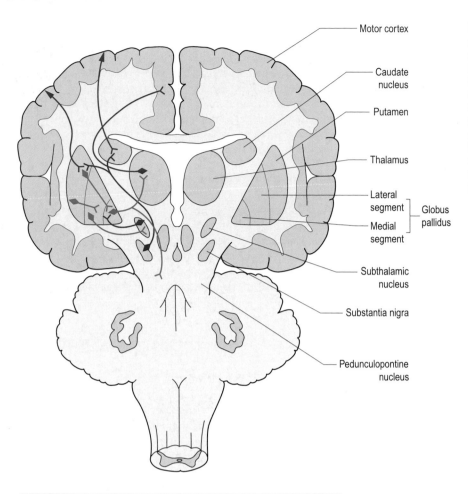

Motor cortex

Caudate nucleus

Putamen

Thalamus

Lateral segment
Medial segment
} Globus pallidus

Subthalamic nucleus

Substantia nigra

Pedunculopontine nucleus

Fig. 14.5 **Schematic diagram illustrating the principal connections of the corpus striatum and related nuclei.** Afferents to the striatum from the intralaminar thalamic nuclei and raphe nuclei have been omitted. For the sake of clarity, all efferents from the basal ganglia system are shown to originate from the medial segment of the globus pallidus, those from the pars reticulata of the substantia nigra being omitted. Similarly, efferents from the striatum are shown to originate only from the putamen and not from the caudate nucleus. (Red, glutamatergic pathways; green, GABAergic pathways; purple, dopaminergic pathway.)

Connections of the striatum

- The caudate nucleus and putamen are the 'input' regions of the corpus striatum.
- They receive afferents from the cerebral cortex, intralaminar thalamic nuclei and the pars compacta of the substantia nigra.
- Efferent fibres are directed to the globus pallidus and the pars reticulata of the substantia nigra.

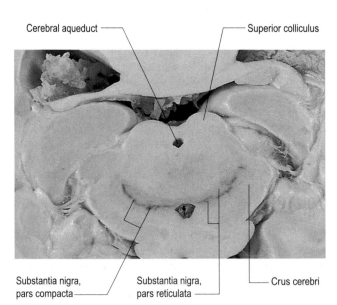

Cerebral aqueduct

Superior colliculus

Substantia nigra, pars compacta

Substantia nigra, pars reticulata

Crus cerebri

Fig. 14.6 **Transverse section through the midbrain showing the substantia nigra.**

Striatal efferents

The efferent projections of the striatum are directed principally to the two segments of the globus pallidus and to the pars reticulata of the substantia nigra (**striatopallidal** and **striatonigral fibres**, respectively). The cells of origin are so-called medium spiny neurones, which make up the vast majority of striatal nerve cells. Generally speaking, although there is some collateralisation, separate populations of neurones project to each of the three output targets (Fig. 14.5). These projections are inhibitory upon pallidal and nigral neurones and utilise GABA as their primary transmitter. In addition, a number of neuropeptides are co-localised in these efferent neurones. The cells that project to the medial segment of the globus pallidus and the substantia nigra contain both **substance P** and **dynorphin**. The projection to the lateral segment of the globus pallidus contains **met-enkephalin**.

Connections of the globus pallidus

The two segments of the globus pallidus have similar afferent connections but substantially different efferent projections. The medial segment of the globus pallidus is very similar in structure and function to the pars reticulata of the substantia nigra, from which it is separated by the internal capsule. Together, the medial pallidum and pars reticulata of the substantia nigra are regarded as the 'output' portion of the basal ganglia, since they are the origin of the majority of basal ganglia efferent fibres that project to other levels of the neuraxis.

Pallidal afferents

Pallidal afferents arise principally from the striatum and from the subthalamic nucleus. Striatopallidal fibres are of

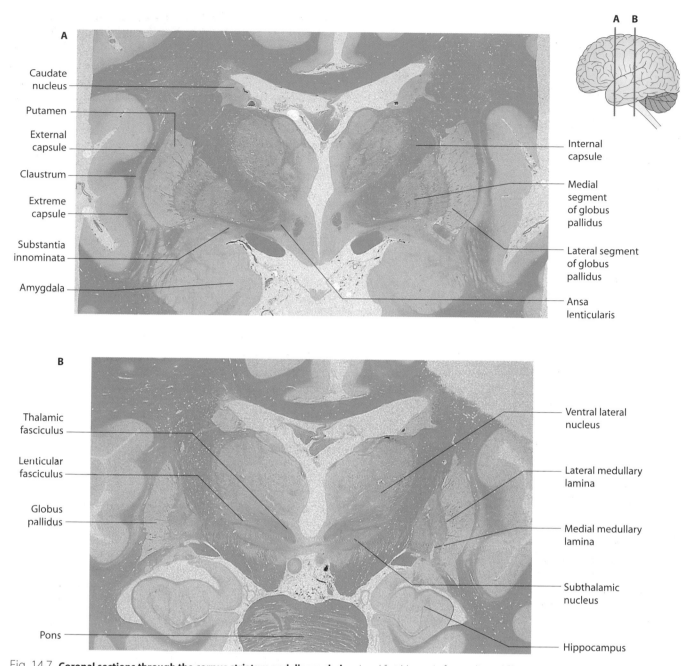

Fig. 14.7 **Coronal sections through the corpus striatum and diencephalon.** Luxol fast blue stain for myelinated fibres.

two types, as previously noted, originating from different populations of striatal neurones. Both utilise GABA as their primary transmitter. In addition, each contains characteristic peptide cotransmitters; fibres projecting to the lateral pallidal segment contain enkephalin, while those projecting to the medial pallidum contain substance P and dynorphin.

The **subthalamopallidal projection** originates in the subthalamic nucleus of the caudal diencephalon (Figs 14.7 and 14.8). This small structure is located beneath the thalamus, lying against the medial surface of the internal capsule. In coronal sections, it has the appearance of a biconvex lens. Subthalamopallidal fibres pass laterally through the internal capsule, contributing to a fibre system known as the **subthalamic fasciculus** (Fig. 14.8), and terminate in both segments of the globus pallidus, although termination is more dense in the medial segment.

The subthalamopallidal pathway is excitatory to pallidal neurones, using glutamic acid as its transmitter. The subthalamic nucleus also sends similar fibres to the pars reticulata of the substantia nigra, the other 'output' part of the basal ganglia system. The subthalamopallidal and subthalamonigral pathways have a pivotal role in the normal function of the basal ganglia and in the pathophysiology of basal ganglia disorders.

Pallidal efferents

The two pallidal segments have different efferent projections. The lateral segment projects principally to the subthalamic nucleus. Pallidosubthalamic fibres pass medially through the internal capsule in the subthalamic fasciculus. This projection is inhibitory and uses GABA as its transmitter. The medial segment of the globus pallidus, together with the pars reticulata of the substantia nigra, projects primarily to the thalamus (ventral lateral, ventral anterior and centromedian nuclei), with a smaller projection to the brain stem tegmentum. These output neurones are inhibitory and utilise GABA as their transmitter.

Pallidothalamic fibres take one of two routes to reach their target (Fig. 14.8). Some fibres pass round the anterior margin of the internal capsule as the **ansa lenticularis**, while others pass through the internal capsule as the **lenticular fasciculus**. The fibres continue to course medially and then loop dorsally and laterally as the **thalamic fasciculus** to enter the thalamus from its ventral aspect. In following this trajectory, the fibres circumnavigate a cellular region of the subthalamus known as the **zona incerta**, which lies between the thalamus and the subthalamic nucleus.

Pallidothalamic fibres constitute the main outflow from the basal ganglia. Their thalamic target nuclei (ventral anterior and ventral lateral), in turn, project excitatory fibres to the motor regions of the frontal lobe, principally the primary motor and supplementary motor cortices. A smaller contingent of medial pallidal efferent fibres passes caudally to terminate in the brain stem tegmentum in the **nucleus tegmenti pedunculopontinus** (pedunculopontine nucleus), which lies at the boundary between midbrain and pons, surrounding the superior cerebellar peduncle (Figs 14.5 and 13.12). This region has been termed the **mesencephalic locomotor region** in lower mammals, since it is involved in the regulation of quadrupedal progression.

The pars reticulata of the substantia nigra is regarded as a homologue of the medial segment of the globus pallidus and to occupy a similar status as the origin of basal ganglia output. Like the medial pallidum, the pars reticulata receives fibres from the striatum and the subthalamic nucleus. The projection from the striatum is somatotopically organised, both in the pallidum and nigra, such that pallidal neurones are associated primarily with limb movements, whereas nigral cells control the axial musculature, including the extraocular muscles. As already noted, efferents from the medial pallidum project to the ventral anterior, ventral lateral and centromedian thalamic nuclei and to the

pedunculopontine nucleus. Efferents of the pars reticulata of the substantia nigra also pass to a subregion of the ventral lateral thalamus, to the superior colliculus and to the brain stem reticular formation (including the pedunculopontine nucleus).

Normal functions of the basal ganglia

The basal ganglia are sometimes referred to as components of the so-called 'extrapyramidal motor system'. This term was coined to distinguish the symptoms seen clinically in diseases of the basal ganglia and related structures such as the substantia nigra and subthalamic nucleus, from those observed following stroke in the internal capsule, the latter being thought to be caused by destruction of the pyramidal tract. As understanding of the functional anatomy of the motor system has increased, it has become apparent both that the pyramidal and extrapyramidal systems are

> ## Connections of the globus pallidus
>
> - The globus pallidus consists of two segments: medial (internal) and lateral (external).
> - The medial segment shares many similarities with the pars reticulata of the substantia nigra and, together, these two structures are regarded as the 'output' regions of the corpus striatum.
> - The globus pallidus receives afferent fibres from the striatum and the subthalamic nucleus.
> - The lateral segment of the globus pallidus projects to the subthalamic nucleus.
> - The medial segment of the globus pallidus projects primarily to the thalamus (ventral anterior, ventral lateral and centromedian nuclei).
> - The thalamus in turn sends fibres to the motor areas of the frontal lobe.

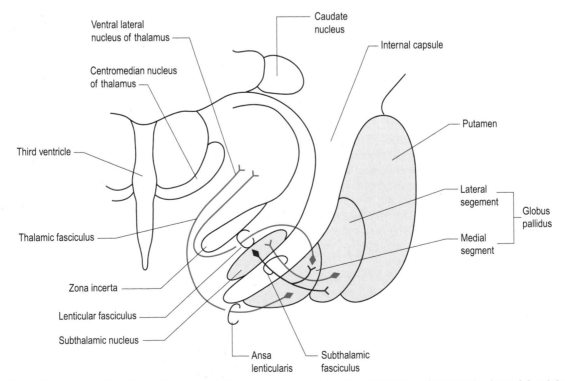

Fig. 14.8 **Schematic coronal section through the corpus striatum and diencephalon illustrating the efferent projections of the globus pallidus.**

intimately related rather than separate, and also that so-called pyramidal signs are not all attributable to dysfunction of the pyramidal tract itself. The term extrapyramidal is, therefore, somewhat outdated but is still in widespread use.

Current concepts of the role of the basal ganglia consider that their function is to facilitate behaviour and movements that are required and appropriate in any particular context and to inhibit unwanted or inappropriate movements. How this might be achieved can be explained with reference to the internal connections of the basal ganglia (Fig. 14.5).

When a movement is initiated from the cerebral cortex, impulses discharge not only through corticospinal and corticobulbar pathways but also through the corticostriatal projection to the neostriatum. These glutamatergic fibres cause excitation of striatal neurones. The striatum has two routes by which it is able to control the activity of basal ganglia output neurones in the medial segment of the globus pallidus or the pars reticulata of the substantia nigra. The first of these is the so-called 'direct pathway', consisting of striatopallidal and striatonigral neurones which directly inhibit medial pallidal or pars reticulata neurones. This mechanism has been shown to operate in experimental electrophysiological studies in primates, where basal ganglia output neurones associated with a particular body part or muscle group show a pause in their action potential discharge during movement of that region. (This has been shown in the medial pallidum for limb movements and in the substantia nigra, pars reticulata for eye movements.) Since medial pallidal and pars reticulata output neurones are themselves inhibitory, this leads to disinhibition of target neurones, including those of the motor thalamus. The resulting increase in the activity of thalamic neurones causes excitation of the cells of the cerebral cortex. The effect of activation of the direct pathway is, therefore, to support or facilitate ongoing movements.

The second route by which striatal neurones can influence the output of the basal ganglia is the so-called 'indirect pathway', via the subthalamic nucleus. Efferents from the striatum terminate in the lateral pallidal segment and their activation induces inhibition of lateral pallidal neurones. The principal efferent projection of the lateral pallidum is to the subthalamic nucleus which, therefore, becomes disinhibited. The resultant increase in discharge of subthalamic neurones causes activation of medial pallidal and nigral neurones and, in turn, inhibition of thalamic and cortical cells. This has the effect of inhibiting unwanted movements.

Fig. 14.9 **Schematic diagram illustrating how activities in basal ganglia and related nuclei become disordered in parkinsonism and chorea.** Overactive pathways are shown by bold lines; underactive pathways are shown by interrupted lines. Pathways coloured as in Figure 14.5.

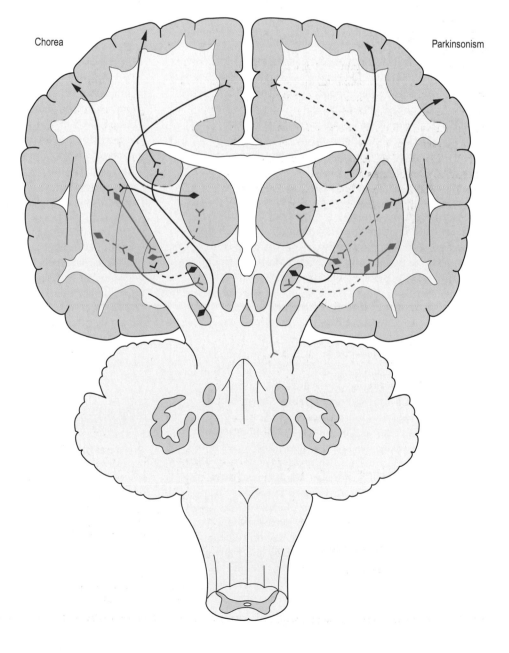

Pathophysiology of basal ganglia disorders

Studies on the post-mortem brains of patients with **Parkinson's disease** and experimental animal studies have provided insight into the pathophysiological mechanisms that underlie the appearance of parkinsonian symptoms (Fig. 14.9). Normally, dopamine appears to exert an excitatory influence upon striatal neurones of the 'direct' projection to the medial pallidal segment, and an inhibitory effect upon neurones of the 'indirect' pathway that projects to the lateral pallidal segment. Loss of striatal dopamine, therefore, causes abnormal underactivity of the direct pathway and disinhibition of medial pallidal neurones. Simultaneously, overactivity of the indirect projection leads to inhibition of lateral pallidal neurones, disinhibition of the subthalamic nucleus, and thus excessive excitatory drive of medial pallidal cells. Changes in both the direct and indirect pathways, thus, compound to exacerbate the abnormal overactivity of medial pallidal output cells, inducing akinesia.

The archetypal basal ganglia disease in which excessive, unwanted, abnormal movements (dyskinesias) occur is **Huntington's disease**. Within the striatum, there is particular attrition of the cells that project to the lateral segment of the globus pallidus (the 'indirect' projection), at

Basal ganglia syndromes

Unilateral basal ganglia lesions produce their effects on the opposite (contralateral) side of the body, as is the case with cerebral hemisphere lesions but distinct from cerebellar disorders. Basal ganglia dysfunction does not cause paralysis, sensory loss or ataxia, but leads to **abnormal motor control**, **alterations in muscular tone** and the emergence of abnormal, involuntary movements, or **dyskinesias**.

Abnormal motor control may consist of slowness of movement (**bradykinesia**) or poverty of movement (**hypokinesia, akinesia**). The initiation, sequencing and cessation of movement are disrupted. Normal posture cannot be maintained and 'associated' limb movements are lost, e.g. arm swinging when walking.

Tone may be increased throughout the range of passive movement (**rigidity**) and the hypertonia may be continuous (plastic) or discontinuous ('cogwheel'). Alternatively, **hypotonia** may occur.

Dyskinesias may be manifest in various ways and describe the abnormal movements, not the underlying disease. **Tremor** is a to-and-fro, sinusoidal movement that may be maximal at rest (resting tremor) or on action (action or postural tremor). **Chorea** is a sequence of rapid, asymmetrical, and fragmented (quasi-purposeful) movements usually affecting the distal limb musculature. **Dystonia** refers to sustained muscular contractions that give rise to abnormal postures or contortions. **Athetosis** consists of slow, sinuous, writhing movements. Sometimes movements share more than one characteristic; hence the term **choreo-athetosis**). **Myoclonus** describes sudden, shock-like movements, which are usually bilateral and especially affect the upper limbs. **Tics** are stereotyped movements, often highly characteristic of the individual, sometimes multiple and frequently influenced by emotional stress.

Basal ganglia diseases

Parkinson's disease is a neurodegenerative disease, usually of the elderly, of unknown cause (idiopathic). It is characterised by akinesia, a flexed posture, rigidity and a resting tremor. The pathological hallmark of Parkinson's disease is degeneration of the dopaminergic neurones of the pars compacta of the substantia nigra, and depletion of striatal dopamine levels (Fig. 14.11). The most effective treatment currently available for the condition is administration of levodopa (L-dopa), the immediate metabolic precursor of dopamine, or dopamine receptor agonists. Levodopa is converted to dopamine and restores normal striatal function, a strategy that can often be used to minimise symptoms for many years. When drug therapy fails, neurosurgical ablation or electrical stimulation of the subthalamic nucleus or the medial segment of the globus pallidus can help the patient.

Huntington's disease is a degenerative disease inherited in an autosomal dominant manner and characterised by chorea and progressive dementia. Pathologically, there is progressive degeneration of the striatum and cerebral cortex. **Hepatolenticular degeneration (Wilson's disease)** is an inherited disorder (autosomal recessive) of copper metabolism. Basal ganglia changes lead to choreo-athetosis and progressive dementia in childhood and youth. **Sydenham's chorea** is now rare but was formerly a common manifestation of rheumatic fever in young females, causing abnormal behaviour and generalised chorea (**St Vitus' dance**).

Levodopa-induced dyskinesia is a complication of the long-term treatment of Parkinson's disease with levodopa, and **tardive dyskinesia** is a long-term complication of the treatment of schizophrenia with neuroleptic drugs. **Hemiballism** is a rare condition characterised by violent choreiform movements of the limbs on one side of the body. It is caused by a lesion, usually of cerebrovascular origin, of the contralateral subthalamic nucleus. **Dystonia** may arise as an inherited disorder of children and is usually generalised. In adults, focal or segmental dystonias affect the arm and hand (writer's cramp), leg, neck (torticollis) or face and mouth (orofacial dyskinesia).

Basal ganglia function

- The basal ganglia historically were referred to as parts of the extrapyramidal motor system to distinguish diseases of this area from those of the pyramidal tract. However, both systems are intimately related.
- The basal ganglia facilitate purposeful behaviour and movement via the direct pathway and inhibit unwanted movements via the indirect pathway.
- Lesions of the basal ganglia produce effects on the contralateral side of the body.
- Diseases of the basal ganglia include Parkinson's disease and Huntington's disease.

least early on in the condition. This leads to disinhibition of lateral pallidal neurones and inhibition of the subthalamic nucleus (Fig. 14.9). Medial pallidal neurones, therefore, become abnormally underactive and unwanted, involuntary movements ensue.

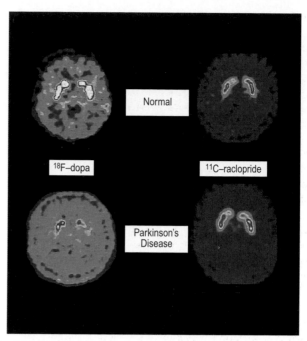

Fig. 14.11 **Four positron emission tomography (PET) scans, representing horizontal sections through the brain (anterior towards the top in each case) at the level of the striatum.** The top scans are from a normal individual and the bottom ones from a patient with Parkinson's disease. The scans on the left were made using the tracer [^{18}F]-dopa. This is taken up by intact dopaminergic nerve terminals and, therefore, acts as an index of the integrity of the nigrostriatal pathway. Note the reduced labelling in the striatum of the parkinsonian patient. The scans on the right were made using the tracer [^{11}C]-raclopride. This binds to dopamine receptors located on striatal neurones that receive input from the nigrostriatal pathway. Note that these receptors remain intact in the parkinsonian patient. (Courtesy of Professor D J Brooks)

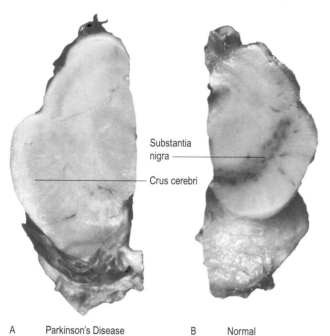

A Parkinson's Disease   B Normal

Fig. 14.10 **Approximately transverse sections through the lateral half of the midbrain, showing degeneration and depigmentation of the substantia nigra, pars compacta in Parkinson's disease.** (Courtesy of Professor D M Mann).

Chapter 15
Visual system

Vision is the most highly developed and versatile of all the sensory modalities and, arguably, the one on which humans are most dependent. The optic nerve and retina develop from the prosencephalic primary brain vesicle and, therefore, are regarded as an outgrowth of the brain itself. Vision commences with the formation of an image of the external world on the photoreceptive **retina**. The retina encodes visual information in the discharge of neurones that project to the brain through the **optic nerve**. Fibres of the optic nerve undergo hemidecussation in the **optic chiasma** and project to the lateral geniculate nucleus of the thalamus. Thalamocortical neurones in turn project to the primary visual cortex of the occipital lobe where visual perception occurs.

The eye

The eyeball, or globe, is approximately spherical in shape (Fig. 15.1). Near its posterior pole emerges the optic nerve. The eyeball may be considered to consist of three concentric layers of tissue, the outermost of which is tough, fibrous and protective. Over most of the globe it forms an opaque white coat, the **sclera**, to which are attached the extraocular muscles. Over the anterior pole of the globe it forms the transparent **cornea**, through which light enters the eye.

Near to the anterior margin of the sclera, two rings of smooth muscle extend into the lumen of the eyeball (Fig. 15.2). The most anterior of these is the **iris**, which has a central aperture, the **pupil**, through which light is admitted to the posterior part of the eye. Some of the muscle fibres of the iris are arranged in a circular fashion, while others are oriented radially. They are under the control of the autonomic nervous system. Circular fibres are innervated by parasympathetic neurones, which act to constrict the pupil and reduce the amount of light falling upon the retina (see p. 104). Radial fibres are innervated by sympathetic neurones to dilate the pupil.

Behind the iris lies the **ciliary body** containing **ciliary muscle**, which receives innervation from the parasympathetic nervous system. The central aperture within the annulus of the ciliary body is occupied by the transparent, biconvex **lens**, which focuses light upon the retina. The lens is held in place by a **suspensory ligament** that is attached to the peripheral margin of the lens and to the ciliary body. Contraction of the ciliary muscle alters the shape and, therefore, the focusing power (focal length) of the lens, a process known as accommodation. The lens and suspensory ligament divide the lumen of the eyeball into an anterior and a posterior part. The anterior part, in front of the lens, contains a thin, watery fluid, known as **aqueous humour**, which is continuously secreted from the ciliary body. It is also reabsorbed into the ciliary body where it accumulates in a small duct, the **canal of Schlemm**,

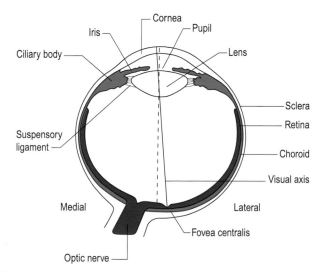

Fig. 15.1 **Schematic drawing of a horizontal section through the right eyeball.**

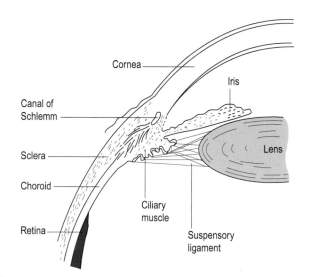

Fig. 15.2 **Schematic drawing of the sclerocorneal junction of the eyeball.**

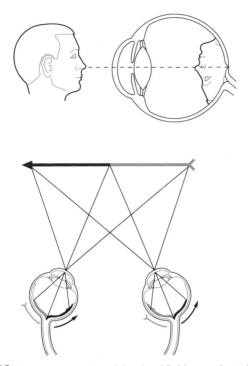

Fig. 15.3 **The representation of the visual field upon the retinae.**

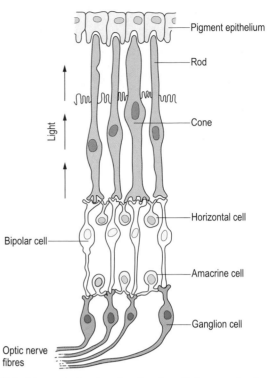

Fig. 15.4 **Schematic drawing showing the cellular organisation of the retina.**

through which it is returned to the venous system. The posterior part of the globe contains a gelatinous material known as **vitreous humour**. Behind the ciliary body, the inner surface of the sclera is lined by the **choroid**, the cells of which contain dark pigment that absorbs light and thus reduces reflection within the eye. Lining the inner surface of the choroid is the photoreceptive retina.

Light passes from objects in the field of vision (**visual field**), through the narrow aperture of the pupil to subtend an image upon the retina. An object in the visual field, upon which attention is focused, subtends an image that is centred near the posterior pole of the eye along the line of the **visual axis** (Fig. 15.1). At this point, which is known as the **fovea centralis**, and the surrounding 1 cm, which is known as the **macula lutea**, the retina is specially modified for maximal visual acuity (resolving power). The basic optical properties of the eye, which may be likened to those of a pinhole camera, dictate that the image so formed is inverted in both lateral and vertical dimensions (Fig. 15.3). Furthermore, objects that lie in the left half of the visual field form an image upon the nasal (right) half of the left retina and the temporal (right) half of the right retina, and vice versa. Medial to the macula is a region where retinal axons accumulate to leave the eye in the optic nerve. This is known as the **optic disc**. Photoreceptors are absent from this region, which is also referred to as the **blind spot**.

Retina

The retina consists of a non-neural and a neural portion. The non-neural part is represented by the **pigment epithelium**, a single layer of light-absorbing, pigmented cells lying adjacent to the choroid (Fig. 15.4). The neural part of the retina contains photoreceptors and neurones as well as neuroglia and a rich capillary network. The photoreceptive cells lie deepest within the retina and interdigitate with the pigment epithelium. Light entering the eye, therefore, passes

through, and is refracted and partially absorbed by, these additional elements before reaching the photoreceptors. By means of a series of photochemical reactions and physicochemical changes, retinal photoreceptors transduce light energy into electrical energy (changes in membrane potential). Retinal photoreceptors are of two types, **rods** and **cones**, of which the rods are about 20 times more numerous. These cells share many structural similarities but have important functional distinctions. Rods are exquisitely sensitive to light. They are particularly important for vision in dim lighting conditions. Cones are responsible for colour vision and, because of their arrangement and neuronal connections, they confer high visual acuity.

Rods and cones are heterogeneously distributed across the retina. Rods greatly predominate in the peripheral parts of the retina but their relative numbers decrease towards the macula, where cones are more abundant. At the fovea only cones are present. Furthermore, at the fovea the neurones and capillaries, through which light has to pass to reach the photoreceptors, are displaced so that the cones are directly exposed to light. This combination provides for maximal visual acuity.

In addition to photoreceptive cells, the retina contains both the first- and second-order neurones of the central visual pathway (Fig. 15.4). The first-order neurone, or **bipolar cell**, lies entirely within the retina, while the axon of the second-order neurone, or **ganglion cell**, forms the optic nerve. Information is transferred from photoreceptors to bipolar cells and then to ganglion cells, with greater convergence for rods than for cones. The retina also contains interneurones known as horizontal cells and amacrine cells. These modulate transmission between photoreceptors and bipolar cells, and between bipolar cells and ganglion cells, respectively.

The eye

- Objects in one lateral half of the visual field form images on the nasal half of the ipsilateral retina and the temporal half of the contralateral retina.
- The retina contains photoreceptors (rods and cones), first-order sensory neurones (bipolar cells) and second-order neurones (ganglion cells).
- The axons of retinal ganglion cells accumulate at the optic disc (blind spot) and pass into the optic nerve.

The central visual pathway

The axons of retinal ganglion cells assemble at the optic disc and pass into the optic nerve, which enters the cranial cavity through the optic canal. The two optic nerves converge to form the **optic chiasma** on the base of the brain (Fig. 15.5). The chiasma lies immediately rostral to the tuber cinereum of the hypothalamus and between the terminating internal carotid arteries. In the chiasma, axons derived from the nasal portions of the two retinae decussate and pass into the contralateral **optic tract**, while those from the temporal hemiretinae remain ipsilateral. The optic tracts diverge away

from the chiasma and pass round the cerebral peduncle to terminate mainly in the lateral geniculate nucleus (within the lateral geniculate body) of the thalamus. A relatively small number of fibres leave the optic nerve, before reaching the lateral geniculate nucleus, to terminate in the **pretectal area** and the superior colliculus. These fibres are involved in mediation of the pupillary light reflex (Chapter 10). From the lateral geniculate nucleus, third-order thalamocortical neurones project through the retrolenticular part of the internal capsule and form the **optic radiation**, which terminates in the primary visual cortex of the occipital lobe. The primary visual cortex is located predominantly on the medial surface of the hemisphere in the region above and below the calcarine sulcus. Surrounding this area, the rest of the occipital lobe constitutes the visual association cortex. It is concerned with interpretation of visual images, recognition, depth perception and colour vision.

There is a precise point-to-point relationship between the retina and the visual cortex. Because of the importance of the macula in vision, it is represented by disproportionately large volumes (relative to its size) of the lateral geniculate nucleus and the visual cortex. Within the visual cortex the macula is represented most posteriorly, in the region of the occipital pole.

As previously noted, objects in either half (left or right) of the visual field produce images upon the nasal hemiretina of the ipsilateral eye and the temporal hemiretina of the contralateral eye (Fig. 15.5). Each optic nerve, therefore, carries information concerning both halves of the visual field. Because of the decussation of fibres from the nasal hemiretinae at the optic chiasma, however, each optic tract, lateral geniculate nucleus and visual cortex receives information relating only to the contralateral half of the visual field. This combination of the images from both eyes is necessary for stereoscopic vision (depth perception). The upper half of the visual field forms images upon the lower halves of the retinae, the lower visual field upon the upper hemiretinae. As thalamocortical fibres leave the lateral geniculate nucleus they pass around the lateral ventricle, those representing the lower part of the visual field coursing superiorly to terminate in the visual cortex above the calcarine sulcus. Those which represent the upper part of the visual field sweep into the temporal lobe (**Meyer's loop,** Fig. 15.6) before terminating below the calcarine sulcus.

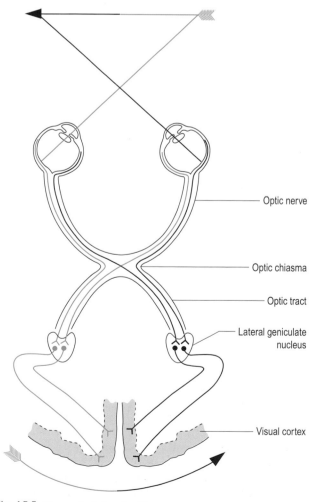

Optic nerve

Optic chiasma

Optic tract

Lateral geniculate nucleus

Visual cortex

Fig. 15.5 **The central visual pathway.**

The central visual pathway

- At the optic chiasma, axons from the nasal halves of the two retinae decussate and pass into the contralateral optic tract.
- The optic tract contains axons that carry information relating to the contralateral half of the field of vision.
- Optic tract fibres end in the lateral geniculate nucleus of the thalamus.
- Third-order visual fibres from the lateral geniculate nucleus pass through the retrolenticular part of the internal capsule and the visual radiations to terminate in the primary visual cortex.
- The primary visual cortex is located above and below the calcarine sulcus of the occipital lobe.
- The rest of the occipital lobe constitutes the visual association area.

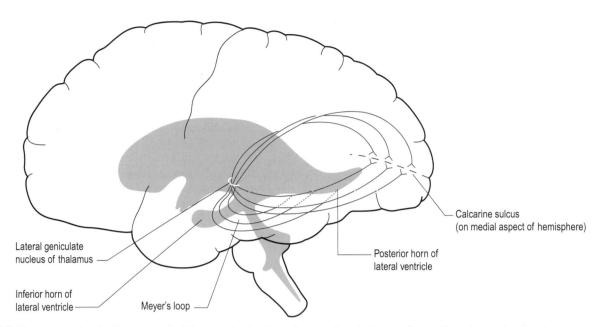

Lateral geniculate
nucleus of thalamus

Inferior horn of
lateral ventricle

Meyer's loop

Calcarine sulcus
(on medial aspect of hemisphere)

Posterior horn of
lateral ventricle

Fig. 15.6 **The course taken by thalamocortical fibres projecting from the lateral geniculate nucleus to the primary visual cortex.**

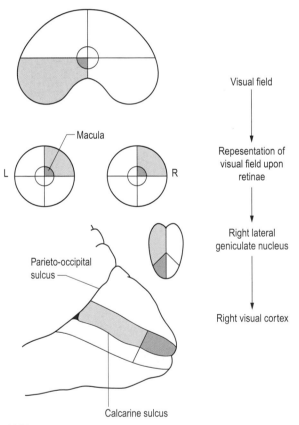

Macula

L

R

Parieto-occipital
sulcus

Calcarine sulcus

Visual field

↓

Repesentation of
visual field upon
retinae

↓

Right lateral
geniculate nucleus

↓

Right visual cortex

Fig. 15.7 **A representation of the left half of the visual field at the various levels of the visual pathway.**

The visual field can be considered (Fig. 15.7) as comprising four quadrants (left/right, upper/lower), each projecting to its own quadrant of the primary visual cortex (left/right hemispheres, above/below the calcarine sulcus). There is both lateral and vertical inversion in the projection of the visual field upon the visual cortex such that, for example, the upper left quadrant of the visual field is represented in the lower right quadrant of the visual cortex.

Visual field deficits

Disease of the eyeball (cataract, intraocular haemorrhage, retinal detachment) and disease of the optic nerve (multiple sclerosis and optic nerve tumours) lead to loss of vision in the affected eye (**monocular blindness**). Compression of the optic chiasm by an adjacent pituitary tumour leads to **bitemporal hemianopia**. Vascular and neoplastic lesions of the optic tract, optic radiation or occipital cortex produce a contralateral **homonymous hemianopia** (Fig. 15.8).

Retinitis pigmentosa is an inherited metabolic disorder of the photoreceptor and retinal pigment epithelial cells. There is progressive night blindness, peripheral visual field constriction and pigmentation of the retina visible on ophthalmoscopy.

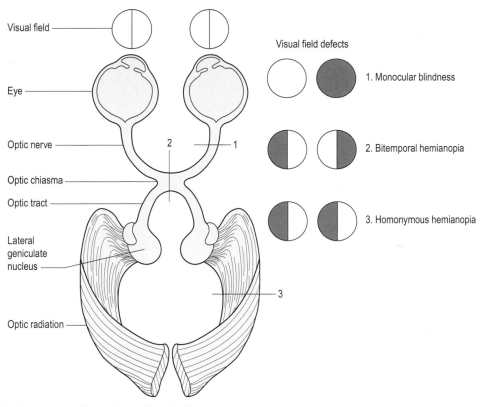

Fig. 15.8 **Visual field deficits produced by lesions of the visual pathway.**

Chapter 16
Hypothalamus, limbic system and olfactory system

In order to survive, there must be continual adaptations to preserve the internal environment of the body (homeostasis). Interoceptor signals from the internal organs and body fluids initiate homeostatic responses; consequently, the internal physical and chemical environment remains balanced and stable. The hypothalamus is the structure responsible for this task.

Exteroceptive information from the outside world dictates behavioural responses in order to achieve individual 'homeostasis' within the physical and social environment. Behaviour is relatively simple and stereotyped in lower animals and directed to satisfying the drives of thirst, hunger, sex and defence, in instinctive repertoires. The limbic system, which is strongly connected to the hypothalamus, is essential for this adaptive behaviour, which includes the ability to learn new responses based on previous experience (memory). The complex and non-stereotyped behaviour of humans is an attempt to preserve the individual within the physical landscape but also within a changing social environment (individual homeostasis). The association areas of the neocortex are capable of analysing exteroceptive information from the environment and other individuals, enabling adaptive personal and social responses. These phylogenetically more recent structures are partly connected to the limbic system.

As a result, the hypothalamus, limbic system and association neocortex act as interfaces in a hierarchical fashion between the internal structure of the individual and the environment. A reminder of this evolutionary ascent in humans is the olfactory system: vital for sensing the environment in lower animals, overwhelmed by visuospatial dominance in humans and intimately related to the limbic system.

Hypothalamus

The hypothalamus is able to integrate interoceptive signals from internal organs and fluid-filled cavities and make appropriate adjustments to the internal environment by virtue of its input and output systems.

The hypothalamic input is circulatory and neural in origin. The circulating blood provides physical (temperature, osmolality), chemical (blood glucose, acid–base state) and hormonal signals of the state of the body, its growth and development and its readiness for action (sex, suckling, defence). Neural signals come from two sources. Firstly, the nucleus solitarius of the medulla projects to the hypothalamus and conveys information collected by the autonomic nervous system concerning the pressure within the smooth-muscled walls of organs (baroreceptors) and the chemical constituents of the fluid-filled cavities (chemoreceptors). Secondly, the state of neural arousal is communicated by two structures in the midbrain: the reticular formation via direct and indirect (via thalamus) routes, and the monoaminergic nuclei via the medial forebrain bundle.

The hypothalamus is capable of generating responses to these stimuli by circulatory and neural means. An intimate relationship with the pituitary gland and privileged access to its circulation (portal system) confers the role of 'orchestrator of the endocrine system' on the hypothalamus, as it directs hormonal synthesis and release. The neural output of the hypothalamus is twofold. Firstly, the autonomic nervous system projects to and controls internal organs, outside conscious control (and, hence, autonomous). Secondly, the hypothalamus is capable of initiating appropriate motor behavioural repertoires of an instinctive kind through its connections with the limbic system and limbic part of the corpus striatum (the nucleus accumbens). Its interconnections with the reticular formation also are capable of influencing the state of wakefulness and sleep.

The hypothalamus has the capability of influencing or overriding more complex adaptive behaviour because of its close links with two important structures: the limbic system and the association cortex of the frontal lobe (orbital part).

Topographical anatomy of the hypothalamus

The hypothalamus is the most ventral part of the diencephalon, lying beneath the thalamus and ventromedial to the subthalamus (Fig. 16.1). It forms the floor and the lower part of the lateral wall of the third ventricle, below the hypothalamic sulcus (Fig. 12.2). On the base of the brain, parts of the hypothalamus can be seen occupying the small area circumscribed by the crura cerebri, optic chiasma and optic tracts (Fig. 12.1). Between the rostral limits of the two crura cerebri, on either side of the midline, lie two distinct, rounded eminences, the **mammillary bodies**, which contain the **mammillary nuclei**. In the midline, immediately caudal to the optic chiasma, lies a small elevated area known as the

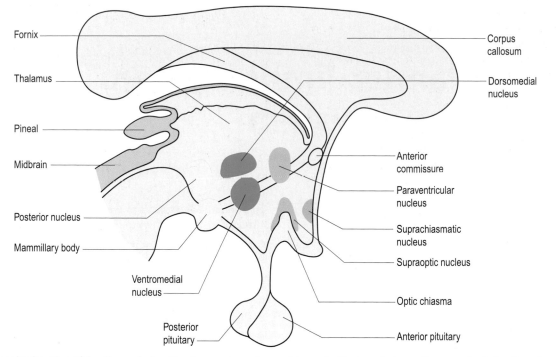

Fig. 16.1 **A sagittal section of the diencephalon.** The diagram shows the medial aspect of the hypothalamus. The approximate location of some of the principal hypothalamic nuclei is shown.

tuber cinereum, from the apex of which extends the thin **infundibulum** (infundibular process), or **pituitary stalk**. This is attached to the **pituitary gland** (**hypophysis**), a pea-sized structure which lies within the sella turcica of the sphenoid bone. The pituitary gland consists of two major, cytologically distinct, parts: the posterior pituitary or **neurohypophysis** and the anterior pituitary or **adenohypophysis** (Figs 16.2 and 16.3). The posterior

pituitary is a neuronal structure, being an expansion of the distal part of the infundibulum. The anterior pituitary is not neural in origin. The two parts are, however, closely linked by the **pituitary** (hypophyseal) **portal system** of vessels (Fig. 16.3), which are derived from the superior hypophyseal artery. Releasing factors, which are synthesised in the hypothalamus, pass to the adenohypophysis through these vessels to control the release of anterior pituitary hormones.

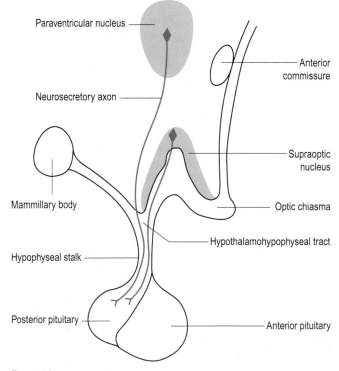

Fig. 16.2 **Supraoptic and paraventricular nuclei projecting to the posterior pituitary via the hypothalamohypophyseal tract.**

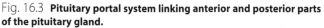

Fig. 16.3 **Pituitary portal system linking anterior and posterior parts of the pituitary gland.**

Hypothalamic nuclei

The hypothalamus consists of many nuclear divisions, only some of which will be described (Fig. 16.1). The region lying medial and ventral to the structures of the subthalamus is known as the **lateral hypothalamus**. It is traversed longitudinally by many fibres, including the medial forebrain bundle. The lateral hypothalamic area is important in the control of food and water intake and is, in part, equivalent to the physiologically defined feeding centre. Lateral hypothalamic lesions cause aphagia and adipsia.

The medial region of the hypothalamus contains various nuclei, only some of which have well-defined functions. Anteriorly lie the supraoptic, paraventricular and suprachiasmatic nuclei. The supraoptic and paraventricular nuclei both produce systemically acting hormones, which are released from the posterior pituitary into the general circulation. The **supraoptic nucleus** produces vasopressin (antidiuretic hormone), which increases water reabsorption by the kidney. The **paraventricular nucleus** synthesises oxytocin. In the female, activation of the paraventricular nucleus, and release of hormone, is induced by suckling. This stimulates milk production by the mammary gland and causes contraction of uterine muscle.

The axons of cells in the supraoptic and paraventricular nuclei pass to the neurohypophysis in the hypothalamohypophyseal tract (Fig. 16.2). The neuroendocrine products are transported in this tract to the neurohypophysis, where they are released into the capillary bed and, thus, reach the general circulation.

The supraoptic nucleus contains osmosensitive neurones that are activated by changes in the osmolality of circulating blood. An increase in osmolality causes release of vasopressin. This acts upon the kidney tubules to increase water reabsorption, thus maintaining water homeostasis.

The hypothalamus also synthesises releasing factors and release-inhibiting factors, which control the release of hormones by the adenohypophysis. The adenohypophysis produces adrenocorticotrophic hormone (ACTH), luteinising hormone (LH), follicle-stimulating hormone (FSH), thyroid-stimulating hormone (TSH), growth hormone and prolactin, which are released into the general circulation. The factors that control them are released from the terminals of hypothalamic neurones into the capillary bed of the pituitary portal system (Fig. 16.3). These vessels, which are intrinsic to

---

Hypothalamus

- The hypothalamus is part of the diencephalon; it is connected to the pituitary gland via the infundibulum.
- The hypothalamus has autonomic, neuroendocrine and limbic functions and is involved in the coordination of homeostatic mechanisms.
- The hypothalamus produces hormones that are released from the posterior pituitary and also releasing factors that control the release of hormones from the anterior pituitary.
- The supraoptic and paraventricular nuclei of the hypothalamus produce vasopressin and oxytocin, respectively.
- Vasopressin and oxytocin are transported to the posterior pituitary in the hypothalamohypophyseal tract.
- The anterior pituitary produces: adrenocorticotrophic hormone, luteinising hormone, follicle-stimulating hormone, thyroid-stimulating hormone, growth hormone and prolactin. Factors that control their secretion are released into the pituitary portal system of the pituitary stalk and carried to the anterior pituitary.
- The lateral hypothalamus and the ventromedial nucleus regulate eating and drinking.

---

the hypophyseal stalk, convey the released agents to the adenohypophysis, where they act upon the hormone-secreting cells. The synthesis of hypothalamic releasing factors is under feedback regulation by hormones produced by target organs.

The **suprachiasmatic nucleus** is concerned with the control of diurnal rhythms and the sleep/waking cycle. It receives some afferent fibres directly from the retina.

More caudally, dorsomedial and ventromedial nuclei lie deep to the lateral wall of the third ventricle. The **ventromedial nucleus**, like the lateral hypothalamus, is concerned with the control of food and fluid intake. The ventromedial nucleus is equated with the physiologically defined satiety centre and lesions of this region cause abnormally increased food intake. In the most caudal part of the hypothalamus lie the posterior nucleus and the **medial mammillary nucleus**, the latter being located within the mammillary body. The mammillary body is part of the limbic system, receiving afferents from the hippocampus and projecting to the anterior nuclei of the thalamus and the brain stem.

The hypothalamus is the brain centre for regulation of the autonomic nervous system. Generally, activation of the posterior hypothalamic domain is associated with sympathetic responses, whereas activation of the anterior hypothalamus is associated with parasympathetic activity.

Limbic system

The limbic system earns its title from its position on the medial rim of the brain (*le grand lobe limbique*). It consists of a number of structures with complex and often looped connections that all ultimately project into the hypothalamus (Fig. 16.4). The powerful input to the limbic system from the neocortical association areas links complex 'goal-directed' behaviour to more primitive, instinctive behaviour and internal homeostasis in a cascade of neural connections (Figs 16.5 and 16.6). In a simplified way, we may conceive of information from the outside world collected in

---

Tumours of the hypothalamus and pituitary gland

Tumours and other diseases of the hypothalamus and associated pituitary gland lead to under- or overproduction of circulating hormones. These, in turn, produce disorders of growth (**dwarfism**, **gigantism** and **acromegaly**), sexual function (**precocious puberty**, **hypogonadism**), body water control (**diabetes insipidus** and **pathological drinking**), eating (**obesity** and **bulimia**) and adrenal cortical control (**Cushing's disease** and **adrenal insufficiency**). Since the pituitary gland is closely adjacent to the optic chiasma, tumours of the gland (**pituitary adenomas**) may lead to bitemporal visual field loss.

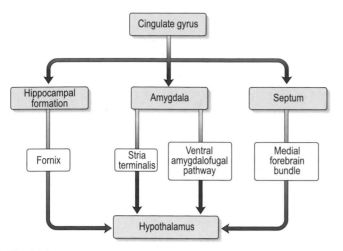

Fig. 16.4 **The principal parts of the limbic system and their relationship with the hypothalamus.**

modality-specific ways (e.g. vision, hearing and touch) and refined in the parieto-occipital association areas (perceptuospatial function). This information is then conveyed to the frontal association areas involved in planned behaviour (regulation) and also to the inferior temporal association areas, where information can reach supramodal status and meaning (semantic processing). Entry of information into the limbic system is either directly to the amygdala, or indirectly to the hippocampal formation, via the entorhinal area. The amygdala appears to provide an affective connotation to experience and especially that relevant to social stimuli. Perhaps affect is an evolutionary development from more primitive 'feelings', derived from the sensory autonomic input from bodily organs into the hypothalamus. The informational flow into the hippocampal formation permits a link to previous experience since the hippocampal formation is essential to remembering and learning (memory).

The limbic system is able to influence motor responses, appropriate to its informational analyses, through projections to the nucleus accumbens, which forms part of the basal ganglia.

Amygdala

The amygdala lies near the temporal pole, between the inferior horn of the lateral ventricle and the lentiform nucleus (Fig. 16.7 and Fig. 13.8). It receives afferents from the inferior temporal association cortex, the septum and the olfactory tract. In addition it receives catecholamine- and serotonin-containing projections from the brain stem in the medial forebrain bundle. The principal efferent projection from the amygdala is the stria terminalis, which runs in the wall of the lateral ventricle, following the curvature of the caudate nucleus, to terminate ultimately in the hypothalamus. The ventral amygdalofugal path also projects to the hypothalamus.

Septum

The septum, or septal region, lies beneath the rostral part of the corpus callosum (Fig. 16.7). It interconnects with the amygdala and projects to the hypothalamus via the medial forebrain bundle. The septum also connects to the monoaminergic nuclei in the brain stem. It does so via fibres that project to the **habenular nuclei** of the diencephalon and constitute the **stria medullaris thalami**. The habenular nuclei in turn project, via the fasciculus retroflexus, to the **interpeduncular nuclei**, which project to the brain stem as well as the hypothalamus. In this way, two major pathways link the septum, the hypothalamus and the monoaminergic nuclei of the brain stem.

Hippocampal formation

The hippocampal formation consists of the hippocampus itself, the dentate gyrus and parts of the parahippocampal gyrus. The **hippocampus** is formed by an infolding of the inferomedial part of the temporal lobe into the lateral ventricle, along the line of the choroid fissure (Fig. 16.8 and

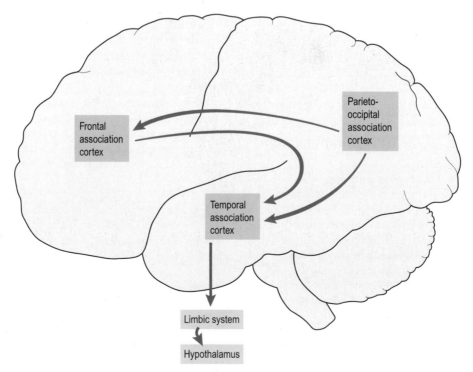

Fig. 16.5 **The link between associative areas of neocortex, the limbic system and the hypothalamus.**

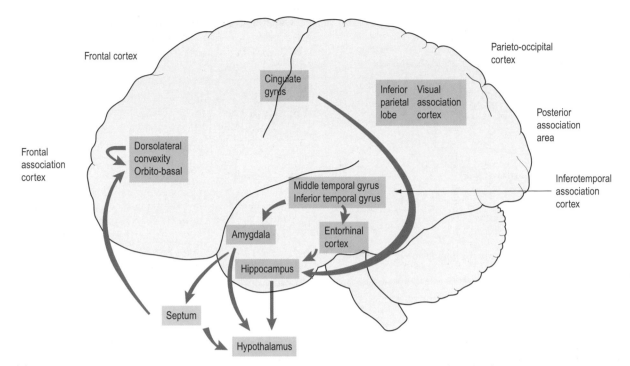

Fig. 16.6 **The interconnections between associative neocortical regions and the component parts of the limbic system.**

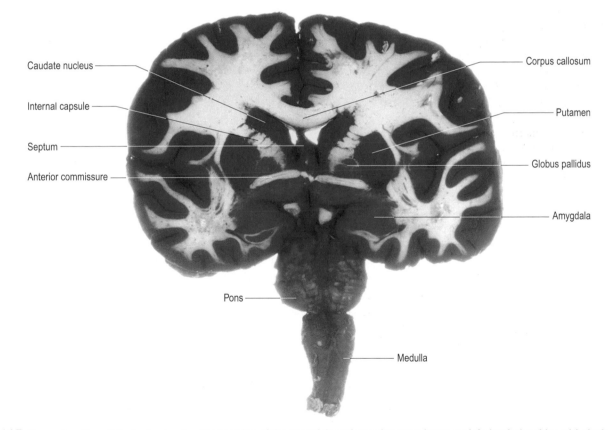

Fig. 16.7 **Coronal section of the brain showing the location of the amygdala and anterior commissure and their relationships with the basal ganglia.** Mulligan's stain (see also Fig. 1.5).

Figs 13.8–13.12). The **dentate gyrus** lies between the parahippocampal gyrus and the hippocampus.

The hippocampal formation receives afferents principally from the inferior temporal cortex via the entorhinal area of the temporal lobe. It also receives fibres from the contralateral entorhinal area and hippocampus via the fornix

system and hippocampal commissure. The principal efferent pathway from the hippocampus is the **fornix** (Figs 12.2, 13.2, 13.7–13.12, Figs 16.9 and 16.10). The fornix is a prominent C-shaped fascicle of fibres that links the hippocampus with the mammillary body of the hypothalamus. Efferent fibres converge on the ventricular surface of the hippocampus as

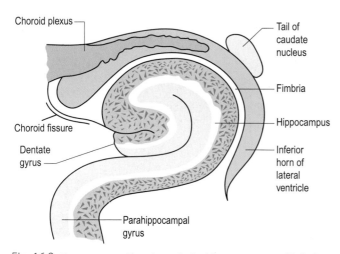

Fig. 16.8 **Transverse section through the hippocampus and inferior horn of the lateral ventricle.**

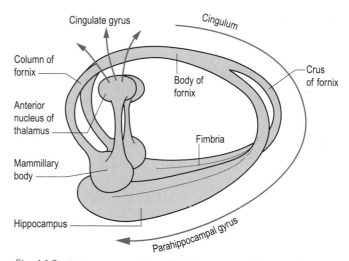

Fig. 16.9 **The interconnection of limbic structures that constitute the Papez circuit.**

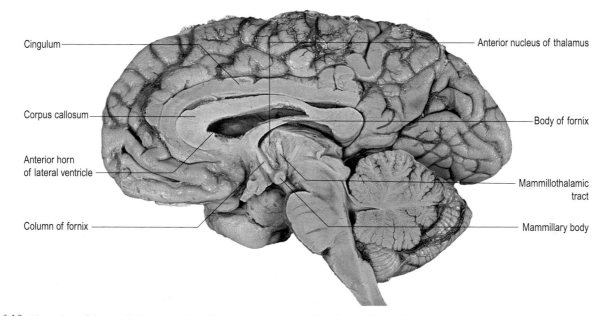

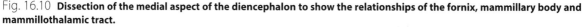

Fig. 16.10 **Dissection of the medial aspect of the diencephalon to show the relationships of the fornix, mammillary body and mammillothalamic tract.**

the **fimbria**. This passes posteriorly and superiorly to become continuous with the crus of the fornix, which then curves forward beneath the splenium of the corpus callosum (Fig. 16.11). The two crura unite in the midline, beneath the corpus callosum, to form the body of the fornix (Fig. 16.10); some fibres cross to the opposite side through the small hippocampal commissure. As it passes forwards beneath the corpus callosum, the body of the fornix divides into two columns. These curve downwards, forming the anterior border of the interventricular foramen, and enter the hypothalamus, where the majority of fibres terminate in the mammillary body. The mammillary body, in turn, projects to the anterior nuclear group of the thalamus via the mammillothalamic tract and to the brain stem via the mammillotegmental tract. The anterior nuclei of the thalamus have major connections with the cingulate gyrus.

Cingulate gyrus
The cingulate gyrus and the **parahippocampal gyrus** are in continuity with one another around the splenium of the

corpus callosum (Fig. 16.12). The cingulate gyrus projects to the parahippocampal gyrus via the fibres of the cingulum (Chapter 13). The principal structures of the limbic system are thus linked by a series of connections, which constitute the **Papez circuit** (Figs 16.9 and 16.10).

Limbic system

- The amygdala is located near to the temporal pole. It receives projections from the olfactory system and the temporal cortex, and has reciprocal connections with the septum.
- The hippocampal formation is made up of the hippocampus, dentate gyrus and parahippocampal gyrus of the temporal lobe. It receives fibres from the entorhinal cortex and projects via the fornix to the mammillary body of the hypothalamus.
- The principal components of the limbic system are interconnected in the Papez circuit.

Head of caudate nucleus ——— Anterior horn of lateral ventricle

Crus of fornix ——— Thalamus

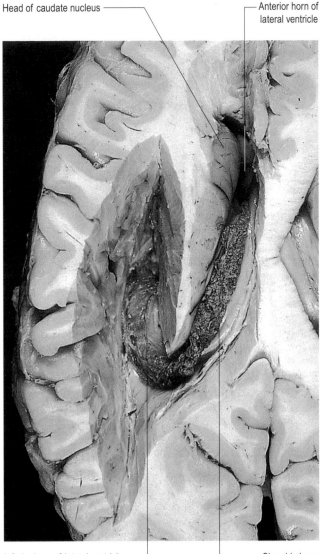

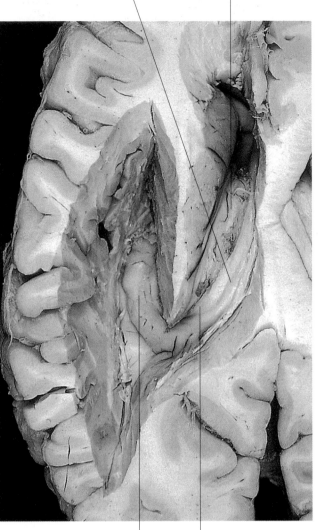

Inferior horn of lateral ventricle ——— Choroid plexus

A

Hippocampus ——— Fimbria

B

Fig. 16.11 **The hippocampus–fimbria–fornix system.** The brain is viewed from above. The cerebral cortex and white matter, including the corpus callosum, have been removed to reveal the lateral ventricle and its contents. **(A)** Choroid plexus of lateral ventricle intact; **(B)** Choroid plexus removed.

Corpus callosum ———

——— Cingulate gyrus

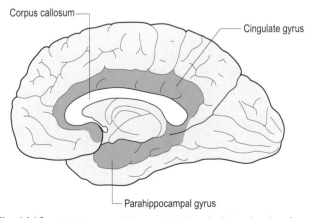

——— Parahippocampal gyrus

Fig. 16.12 **Medial aspect of the cerebral hemisphere showing the relationship between the cingulate gyrus and parahippocampal gyrus.**

Limbic lobe disorders

Alcohol abuse, in a setting of dietary deficiency of thiamine, leads to capillary haemorrhages in the upper brain stem and limbic structures. The patient falls into confusion and coma (**Wernicke's encephalopathy**). Partial recovery may occur, with failure to remember previous experience (retrograde amnesia) or to learn new facts (anterograde amnesia). This is known as **Korsakoff's psychosis**. A similar amnesic syndrome occurs when bilateral, surgical temporal lobectomy incorporates the hippocampal formations.

Temporal lobe or **complex partial seizures** arising close to the amygdala and hippocampi can lead to complex experiences of smell, mood and memory. The states of disordered thinking, hallucinations and strange or violent behaviour can mimic schizophrenia. Surgical ablation of the amygdala has eliminated uncontrollable rage reactions in some psychotic patients.

Olfactory system

Olfactory receptors are specialised, ciliated nerve cells that lie in the olfactory epithelium of the nasal cavity. Their axons assemble into numerous small fascicles (the true olfactory nerves) that enter the cranial cavity through the foramina of the **cribriform plate** of the ethmoid bone (Fig. 5.1) and then attach to the **olfactory bulb** on the inferior surface of the frontal lobe (Fig. 16.13 and Fig. 10.1). Preliminary processing of olfactory information occurs within the olfactory bulb, which contains interneurones and large **mitral cells**; axons from the latter leave the bulb in the olfactory tract.

The olfactory tract passes backwards on the basal surface of the frontal lobe and, just before reaching the level of the optic chiasma, most olfactory tract fibres are deflected laterally, in the **lateral olfactory stria** (Fig. 16.13). These fibres pass into the depths of the lateral fissure, which they cross to reach the temporal lobe. They terminate mainly in the **primary olfactory cortex** of the **uncus** (Fig. 16.13 and Fig. 13.2), on the inferomedial aspect of the temporal lobe, and in the subjacent amygdala. Adjacent to the uncus, the anterior part of the parahippocampal gyrus, or entorhinal area, constitutes the olfactory association cortex. The primary and association cortices are also collectively referred to as the pyriform cortex and are responsible for the appreciation of olfactory stimuli. The olfactory projection is unique among the sensory systems in that it consists of a sequence of only two neurones between the sensory receptors and cerebral cortex and does not project via the thalamus.

Olfactory system

■ Olfactory nerve fibres terminate in the olfactory bulb.
■ Second-order fibres run in the olfactory tract and terminate in the primary olfactory cortex of the uncus in the temporal lobe.
■ Adjacent to this, the anterior part of the parahippocampal gyrus, or entorhinal cortex, constitutes the olfactory association cortex.

Anosmia

Anosmia follows damage to the olfactory nerves. There is loss not only of the sense of smell but also of the flavour of foods. However, elementary aspects of taste, e.g. sweet, salt, bitter and sour, are preserved. Anosmia frequently follows head trauma and can occur when tumours of the meninges (**meningiomas**) invade the olfactory nerves.

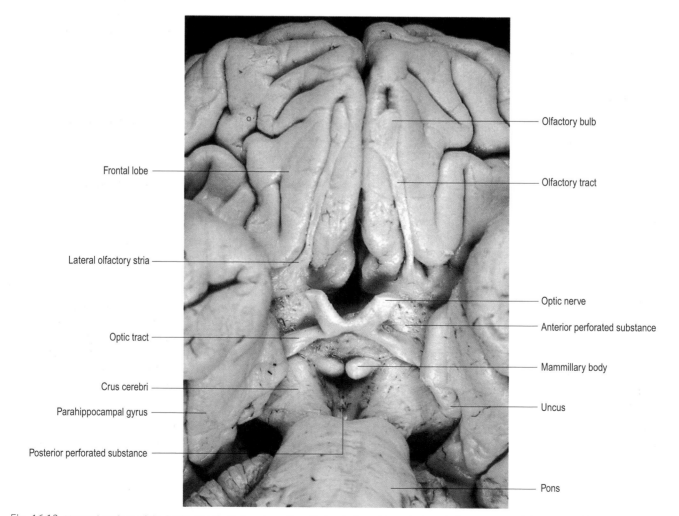

Fig. 16.13 **Ventral surface of the brain.** The illustration shows the olfactory bulb and tract, the lateral olfactory stria and the primary olfactory area of the cerebral cortex (uncus).

Chapter 17
Problem-solving

Introduction

Neuroanatomy is primarily an anatomical rather than a clinical textbook. Neuroanatomy is, however, the foundation of clinical neurological diagnosis. This is because the clinical syndromes, arising from lesions within the neuromuscular system, are determined by the topographical distribution of the lesion, as opposed to its cause. Thus, by combining knowledge of neuroanatomy with the practical skills of the clinical examination, the site of the lesion can be determined with great accuracy at the bedside and before the application of sophisticated investigations. Once the clinical syndrome is defined and the site of the lesion within the nervous system located, it is possible to infer the cause of the lesion by a careful consideration of the evolution of the patient's symptoms, obtained by clinical history-taking. The ultimate diagnosis is reached by applying appropriate investigations in order to clarify the site and cause of the lesion.

In order to exemplify this diagnostic process, a series of problem-solving tasks provide the student, firstly, with sufficient information concerning the clinical neurological findings on examination in order to permit the definition of the syndrome and deduce the localisation of the site of the lesion within the nervous system. Next, the student is given a series of clinical histories, in each case describing the evolution of the patient's symptoms. By combining the information from the clinical examination with the clinical history, the student is asked to suggest the appropriate aetiology corresponding to the case description. The next step is to suggest a critical investigation or series of tests needed to confirm the clinical diagnosis. In the final question, the student is asked to denote the specific disease or diseases giving rise to the clinical symptoms and signs.

All of the information necessary to answer these questions is contained in the text, in the figures or in the clinical boxes marked by a .

Questions

Case 1

Neurological examination

Cranial nerves	Weakness and numbness of the right side of the face.
Motor system	Spasticity and pyramidal weakness of the right arm and leg.
Reflexes	Tendon jerks very brisk on the right; a right extensor plantar response.
Sensation	Loss of sensation in the right arm, trunk and leg.
Coordination	Incoordination of the right limbs.
Mental state	Impairment of speech, comprehension, reading, writing and calculation.

Question
What is the syndrome?

History 1

In the early hours of the morning, having had a heavy drinking session the night before, a 75-year-old man developed the sudden loss of the use of the right side and the power of speech. He had a previous history of ischaemic heart disease, hypertension and diabetes mellitus.

Questions
1. What is the likely cause of the illness?
2. Name the investigation of choice to confirm the diagnosis.
3. Name the disease.

History 2

Over a period of 4 weeks, a 45-year-old man developed progressive weakness of the right side of the body and difficulty in speaking. He had a previous history of two epileptic seizures, occurring within the previous year. On admission to hospital, he was complaining of severe headache, vomiting and drowsiness.

Questions
1. What is the likely cause of the illness?
2. Name the investigation of choice to confirm the diagnosis.
3. Name the disease.

Case 2

Neurological examination

Cranial nerves	Weakness and wasting of the neck muscles.
Motor system	Weakness and wasting of the muscles of the upper arms and legs.
Reflexes	Tendon jerks present; flexor plantar responses.
Sensation	No loss of feeling.
Coordination	A 'waddling' gait.
Mental state	Normal.

Question
What is the syndrome?

History 1

A boy of 12 developed the insidious onset of weakness of the legs with difficulty rising from a chair and climbing steps, followed by gradual weakness of the arms, especially when raised above his head. His father was known to suffer from a similar disorder.

Questions
1. What is the likely cause of the illness?
2. Name the investigation of choice to confirm the diagnosis.
3. Name the disease.

History 2

A 65-year-old female developed the rapid onset of weakness of the arms and legs over the course of a week and then a progressive decline in strength, especially in the proximal limb muscles and accompanied by discomfort and tenderness of the muscles. She had been a lifelong heavy smoker and had also recently developed a productive cough.

Questions
1. What is the likely cause of the illness?
2. Name the investigation of choice to confirm the diagnosis.
3. Name the disease.

Case 3

Neurological examination

Cranial nerves	Intact.
Motor system	Weakness and wasting of the forearms, hands, lower legs and feet; fasciculations of the muscles.
Reflexes	Absent supinator and ankle jerks; flexor plantar responses.
Sensation	Loss of sensation to touch and pinprick below the elbows and the knees; loss of proprioception in the fingers and toes.
Coordination	A limp due to bilateral foot-drop; loss of balance with the eyes closed (positive Romberg's sign).
Mental state	Normal.

Question
What is the syndrome?

History 1

A 50-year-old woman developed the gradual onset of tingling and numbness in the hands and feet over the course of a few months, followed by weakness and wasting of the extremities and loss of balance. She had been generally unwell with loss of weight, despite preserved appetite, and had developed thirst and polyuria.

Questions
1. What is the likely cause of the illness?
2. Name the investigation of choice to confirm the diagnosis.
3. Name the disease.

History 2

A man of 24 years developed the slow onset and progression of tingling numbness and weakness of the extremities with loss of balance over a 5-year period. In retrospect, he had always performed poorly in sport and games and had been told he had a 'funny walk'. His father had been killed in an accident shortly before he was born, but it was thought that his paternal grandfather had had a similar disorder.

Questions
1. What is the likely cause of the illness?
2. Name the investigation of choice to confirm the diagnosis.
3. Name the disease.

Case 4

Neurological examination

Cranial nerves	Intact.
Motor system	Spastic weakness of the legs (paraparesis).
Reflexes	Tendon jerks exaggerated in the legs; bilateral extensor plantar responses; ankle clonus.
Sensation	Loss of feeling to pinprick and touch from the mid-waist downwards; loss of proprioception in the feet.
Coordination	Ataxic gait, worse with the eyes closed (positive Romberg's sign).
Mental state	Normal.

Question
What is the syndrome?

History 1

A 35-year-old Asian male, who had lived in India until travelling to the UK 2 years before, developed pain in the back, radiating into the trunk and waist and, over 2 months, weakness and loss of feeling in the legs, and loss of balance. He had felt generally unwell, with weight-loss and night sweats.

Questions
1. What is the likely cause of the illness?
2. Name the investigation of choice to confirm the diagnosis.
3. Name the disease.

History 2

A 70-year-old man, when standing at a football match, developed sudden pain in the back and immediate paralysis and loss of feeling in the limbs, with incontinence. He was a heavy cigarette smoker and suffered from hypertension.

Questions
1. What is the likely cause of the illness?
2. Name the investigation of choice to confirm the diagnosis.
3. Name the disease.

Case 5

Neurological examination

Cranial nerves	Expressionless face; quiet voice.
Motor system	Rigidity of all four limbs with normal power.
Reflexes	Tendon jerks present; flexor plantar responses.
Sensation	No loss of feeling in the limbs.
Coordination	Stooped posture, shuffling gait, and slow resting tremor of the hands; loss of dexterity.
Mental state	Normal.

Question
What is the syndrome?

History 1
A 65-year-old woman developed the insidious onset, over a year, of slowness of gait, trembling of the hands, loss of dexterity and impairment of writing, in which the script was small.

Questions
1. What is the likely cause of the illness?
2. Name the investigation of choice to confirm the diagnosis.
3. Name the disease.

History 2
A 25-year-old male suffering from schizophrenia, with profound behavioural disturbance and aggression, was admitted to hospital for therapeutic control of his psychosis. He developed slowness and stiffness of the limbs, with a shuffling gait, 10 days after his admission to hospital.

Questions
1. What is the likely cause of the illness?
2. Name the investigation of choice to confirm the diagnosis.
3. Name the disease.

Case 6

Neurological examination

Cranial nerves	Nystagmus; slurred, scanning speech.
Motor system	Power and tone in the limbs normal.
Reflexes	Tendon jerks present; flexor plantar responses.
Sensation	No loss of feeling in the limbs.
Coordination	Impaired coordination of the arms on finger–nose testing. A wide-based ataxic gait.
Mental state	Normal.

Question
What is the syndrome?

History 1
A 55-year-old female developed the insidious onset of a slow and unsteady gait with slurred speech and poor concentration and memory, over a period of 6 months. During that time, she had been noted to gain weight and developed dry skin and hair loss.

Questions
1. What is the likely cause of the illness?
2. Name the investigation of choice to confirm the diagnosis.
3. Name the disease.

History 2
A woman of 25 developed the rapid onset of slurred speech and unsteadiness of the limbs and was incapacitated within 1 week of the onset of symptoms. Two years before, she had suffered rapid loss of vision in the left eye, followed by complete recovery. One year before, she had developed an episode of numbness and tingling of the legs, lasting for a few weeks.

Questions
1. What is the likely cause of the illness?
2. Name the investigation of choice to confirm the diagnosis.
3. Name the disease.

Case 7

Neurological examination

Cranial nerves	Intact.
Motor system	Weakness and wasting; fasciculations of the legs.
Reflexes	Absent knee and ankle jerks; plantar response unobtainable.
Sensation	Loss of sensation to pin, touch and proprioception below the groin.
Coordination	Weak, ataxic gait.
Mental state	Normal.

Question
What is the syndrome?

History 1
A man aged 25 fell from scaffolding on to his back. He developed immediate pain in the low back and, over the course of the next 3 weeks, progressive weakness of the legs, with loss of feeling and incontinence.

Questions
1. What is the likely cause of the illness?
2. Name the investigation of choice to confirm the diagnosis.
3. Name the disease.

History 2
A 65-year-old man developed the rapid onset, over a few days, of pain in the back, and weakness and loss of feeling in the legs, together with incontinence. He had been treated for the previous 2 years for prostatic carcinoma.

Case 8

Optic neuropathy syndrome

History 1
1. Inflammatory disorder
2. MRI imaging of the brain and optic nerves; cerebrospinal fluid examination; visually evoked responses
3. Multiple sclerosis

History 2
1. Extrinsic compression; systemic disease
2. MRI imaging of the brain, optic nerves and chiasma; endocrine investigations of pituitary gland function
3. Pituitary tumour (craniopharyngioma)

Case 9

Amnesic syndrome

History 1
1. Systemic disorder
2. MRI of the brain

3. Wernicke's encephalopathy due to alcoholism, leading to damage to the limbic system and Korsakoff's amnesia

History 2
1. Degenerative disorder
2. MRI of the brain
3. Alzheimer's disease

Case 10

Basal ganglia syndrome

History 1
1. Heredo-degenerative disorder
2. MRI of the brain; genetic DNA analysis
3. Huntington's disease

History 2
1. Systemic disease
2. Serological investigations
3. Sydenham's chorea

Glossary

Acalculia – Inability to calculate.

Accommodation – Act of refocusing the visual image.

Acromegaly – Overgrowth of the skeleton and organs caused by excessive release of growth hormone from a pituitary tumour.

Acuity – Resolving power.

Adenoma – Benign tumour.

Adhesion – Scarring of tissues, fixing them together.

Adipsia – Inability, or loss of desire, to drink.

Aetiology – Relating to the cause of disease.

Afferent – Carrying towards (e.g. cerebellar afferent neurones carry impulses to the cerebellum).

Agnosia – Inability to recognise objects.

Agraphia – Inability to write.

Akinesia – Loss, or slowness, of movement.

Alexia – Inability to read.

Amnesia – Loss of memory.

Anastomosis – Intercommunication between vessels (e.g. circulus arteriosus or circle of Willis).

Aneurysm – Abnormal dilatation of an artery.

Angioma – Congenital swollen collection of blood vessels.

Angiography – Demonstration of the arterial system after injection of an opaque medium.

Anomia – Inability to name objects.

Antidiuretic – An agent that reduces the volume of urine produced by the kidney.

Aphagia – Inability, or loss of desire, to eat.

Aphasia – Loss of ability to use language.

Apraxia – Loss of skilled movements despite preservation of power, sensation and coordination.

Areflexia – Loss of reflexes.

Arthritis – Inflammation of one or more joints.

Astrocyte – A neuroglial cell with fibrous processes.

Ataxia – Loss of ability to coordinate voluntary movements.

Atrophy – Wasting or degeneration.

Axon – The nerve fibre carrying impulses away from the cell body.

Baroreceptor – Neuronal sensory ending that detects changes in arterial blood pressure.

Biopsy – Tissue sample taken from a patient for the diagnosis of disease.

Blood–brain barrier – A selectively permeable barrier between the circulating blood and the brain believed to be formed by astrocytes.

Bulimia – Overeating disorder.

Bradykinesia – Slowness of movement.

Brain stem – The stalk-like portion of the brain connecting the cerebral hemispheres with the spinal cord.

Bulbar palsy – Weakness of tongue, pharynx and larynx resulting from disease of the lower cranial nerves.

Cataract – Opacity of the lens of the eye, leading to deterioration of vision.

Central nervous system – The brain and spinal cord.

Cephalic – Relating to the head.

Cerebrum – The largest, most highly developed part of the brain comprising two cerebral hemispheres.

Cerebrospinal fluid (CSF) – The clear watery fluid that surrounds the brain and spinal cord.

Chemoreceptor – Neuronal sensory ending that detects changes in the chemical composition of circulating blood.

Chiasma – Decussation or crossing over of nerve fibres (e.g. optic chiasma).

Chorea – Involuntary, jerky movements of the face and limbs.

Collateral – A small side branch of a nerve or blood vessel.

Coma – Prolonged and unnatural state of unconsciousness.

Computed tomography (CT) – Imaging technique utilising X-rays to visualise the structure of the nervous system.

Concussion – Loss of consciousness caused by head injury.

Contralateral – Relating to the opposite side.

Contusion – Bruising.

Convulsion – Involuntary contraction or spasm of muscles.

Cordotomy – Neurosurgical procedure to destroy specific pathways in the spinal cord.

Craniopharyngioma – Congenital tumour of the base of the brain.

Craniotomy – Neurosurgical procedure to open the cranial cavity.

Cushing's disease – Overgrowth of the adrenal glands causing excessive release of corticosteroid hormones.

Decussation – Crossing over of nerve fibres from one side of the CNS to the other (e.g. pyramidal decussation).

Dementia – Loss of mental abilities.

Demyelination – Loss of the myelin sheath surrounding neuronal axons.

Dendrite – A short branching process of a neurone that conducts electrical changes to the cell body.

Diabetes insipidus – Failure of the posterior pituitary gland causing reduced release of antidiuretic hormone.

Diabetes mellitus – A disorder of carbohydrate metabolism caused by lack of insulin.

Dysarthria – Inability to pronounce.

Dysphagia – Inability to swallow.

Dysphonia – Inability to produce the voice.

Echocardiography – The use of ultrasound to display the action of the heart.

Efferent – Carrying away from (e.g. striatal efferent fibres carry impulses away from the striatum).

Electroencephalography (EEG) – Technique to detect the surface electrical activity of the brain.

Electromyography – Technique to determine the electrical activity of muscles.

Emetic – Causing nausea and vomiting.

Encephalopathy – Disorder of the brain.

Entrapment neuropathy – Nerve injury caused by compression of a nerve within a tunnel or at a change in direction.

Epilepsy – Paroxysmal attack of disturbed consciousness and sensorimotor function resulting from abnormal electrophysiological discharges of the brain.

Fasciculation – Spontaneous contraction of denervated motor units, visible on inspection.

Fasciculus – Bundle of nerve fibres (e.g. medial longitudinal fasciculus).

Febrile – Refers to raised body temperature (fever).

Fibrillation – Spontaneous contraction of denervated muscle fibres, detected on electromyography.

Foramen – An opening (e.g. foramen magnum).

Ganglion – A collection of nerve cell bodies outside the CNS (e.g. dorsal root ganglion).

General paralysis of the insane (GPI) – Disease of the frontal lobes caused by late neurosyphilis.

Glia – The specialised connective tissue of the CNS comprising oligodendrocytes, astrocytes, ependymal cells and microglia.

Glioma – Tumour derived from glial cells.

Haematoma – Blood clot.

Haemorrhage – Escape of blood from a ruptured blood vessel.

Hallucination – Abnormal perceptual experience.

Hemianopia – Loss of sight affecting one half of the visual field (e.g. bitemporal hemianopia).

Hemiparesis – Weakness of one side of the body.

Hemiplegia – See hemiparesis.

Hepatolenticular degeneration (Wilson's disease) – Inherited disease of copper metabolism affecting the liver and brain.

Herpes zoster – Virus causing shingles (q.v.).

Huntington's disease – Inherited degenerative disease of the brain causing chorea (q.v.) and dementia (q.v.).

Hydrocephalus – Abnormal amount of cerebrospinal fluid within the ventricles of the brain.

Hyperacusis – Increased hearing sensitivity.

Hyperreflexia – Abnormal increase in reflex activity.

Hypertonia – Abnormal increase in muscle tone.

Hypertrophy – Enlargement of tissues.

Hypothyroidism – Underactivity of the thyroid gland causing reduced release of thyroid hormone.

Hypotonia – Abnormal decrease in muscle tone.

Idiopathic – Of unknown cause.

Infarction – Death of tissue resulting from impairment of its circulation.

Intervertebral – Between two vertebrae.

Ipsilateral – Relating to the same side.

Kinaesthesia – Perception of movement.

Lamina – A thin layer (e.g. internal medullary lamina).

Lesion – Site of disease or damage.

Lobectomy – Surgical resection of lobe of the brain.

Lumen – A space or cavity.

Lymphoma – Tumour of the lymphoid system.

Magnetic resonance imaging (MRI) – Technique to image structure that does not employ ionising radiation.

Mastication – The act of chewing.

Miosis – Pupillary constriction.

Meningitis – Inflammation of the meninges.

Meningioma – A tumour arising from the fibrous coverings (meninges) of the brain.

Metastasis – Spread of tumour to distant sites.

Microglia – One of the types of neuroglia (non-nervous cells) of the CNS, having a mainly scavenging function.

Migraine – Paroxysmal headache.

Motor neurone disease – Degenerative disease of upper and lower motor neurones, causing paralysis.

Multiple sclerosis – Immune disease of the CNS, causing relapsing disorder of nervous function.

Muscular dystrophy – Inherited degeneration of muscles, causing progressive paralysis.

Myasthenia gravis – Immune disorder of the neuromuscular junction, causing muscular fatigue.

Myelin – A sheath of protein and phospholipid around the axons of certain neurones.

Myopathy – Disease of muscle.

Narcolepsy – Paroxysmal sleep attacks.

Necrosis – Death of tissue.

Neoplasia – Tumorous overgrowth of tissue.

Neurofibromatosis – Inherited disease causing tumours of meninges, CNS, peripheral nerves and skin.

Neuroma – Tumour derived from nerve cells.

Neurone – A cell specialised to transmit electrical nerve impulses.

Neuropathy – Disease of nerve cells.

Neurosyphilis – Infection of the nervous system by a spirochaete.

Neurotransmitter – A chemical substance released from nerve endings to transmit impulses across synapses.

Nociception – Sensitivity to noxious stimuli.

Nuclcus – Structure within a cell that contains chromosomal DNA; also a collection of nerve cell bodies within the CNS (e.g. dentate nucleus).

Nystagmus – To-and-fro movements of the eyes.

Oedema – Swelling caused by accumulated fluid.

Oligodendrocyte – One of the types of neuroglia; produces the myelin sheath in the CNS.

Oligodendroglioma – Tumour derived from oligodendroglia.

Ophthalmoscopy – Clinical examination of the eye with an ophthalmoscope.

Palsy – Weakness.

Papilloedema – Swelling of the optic nerve(s).

Paraesthesia – Tingling sensations ('pins and needles').

Paralysis – Muscle weakness of varying severity.

Paraphasia – Use of incorrect word.

Paraplegia – Weakness or paralysis of the legs.

Paresis – Muscular weakness.

Parkinson's disease – Disease of the basal ganglia causing akinesia (q.v.), rigidity (q.v.) and tremor (q.v.).

Paroxysm – Sudden attack.

Peripheral nervous system – All parts of the nervous system excluding the brain and spinal cord (CNS).

Photophobia – Intolerance to light.

Plexus – Structure consisting of interwoven nerves (e.g. brachial plexus) or blood vessels (e.g. choroid plexus).

Poliomyelitis – Viral infection of motor neurones of the spinal cord and brain stem.

Positron emission tomography (PET) – Technique for imaging the function of the brain.

Prolapse – Displacement from normal anatomical position.

Proprioception – The detection of position and movement of body parts.

Pseudobulbar palsy – Weakness of the tongue, pharynx and larynx caused by disease of the corticobulbar tracts.

Psychosis – Abnormal mental state with altered precepts (hallucinations) and false ideas (delusions).

Ptosis – Abnormal drooping of the eyelid.

Quadriplegia – Paralysis affecting all four limbs.

Radiculopathy – Disease of the nerve roots.

Resting potential – The electrical potential across the membrane of a cell at rest.

Rheumatic fever – Immune disease of the joints, heart and brain following bacterial infection.

Rigidity – Increased resistance to passive movement of the limbs throughout their range.

Schizophrenia – Disease of the brain causing psychosis (q.v.).

Seizure – Sudden disturbance of consciousness or sensorimotor function.

Shingles – Infection of the ganglia of cranial and spinal nerves by herpes zoster virus (q.v.).

Single photon emission tomography (SPECT) – Technique for imaging the function of the brain.

Somatic – Relating to body parts other than the viscera.

Somatotopic – The orderly representation of body parts in the CNS.

Spasticity – Increased resistance to passive movement of the limbs when muscles are initially stretched.

Spondylosis – Degeneration of the spine.

Stroke – Sudden neurological deficit caused by disease of the circulation to the brain.

Sydenham's chorea – Manifestation of rheumatic fever (q.v.) affecting the basal ganglia and causing involuntary movements.

Synapse – The gap between neurones across which nerve impulses pass by release of a neurotransmitter.

Synaptic vesicles – Structures containing neurotransmitters that release their contents into the synapse on depolarisation of the nerve ending.

Syncope – Fainting attack.

Syndrome – Group of signs and symptoms which characterise a disease.

Syringobulbia – Expanding cavity (syrinx) within the medulla.

Syringomyelia – Expanding cavity within the spinal cord.

Syrinx – An abnormal cavity in the spinal cord.

Thalamotomy – Neurosurgical destruction of part of the thalamus.

Thrombosis – Coagulation of blood in artery or vein.

Tract – An aggregation of nerve cell processes having more or less the same origin and destination (e.g. corticospinal tract).

Tremor – Trembling of head or limbs.

Tumour – A swelling or morbid enlargement; a mass of abnormal tissue resulting from uncontrolled cell growth (neoplasm).

Index